Menopause The Change Challenge

Get Your Hormones Right

Strategies to Beat Insomnia

Cool Hot Flashes

Win Weight Management

and Balance Mood Swings

Freeman Publishing

eBook ISBN 978-1-963333-07-7
Paperback ISBN 978-1-963333-10-7
Hardback ISBN 978-1-963333-11-4
Cover design by 100Covers.com

Table of Contents

Medical Disclaimer: 7
Introduction   9

1. WISDOM IN MENOPAUSE—
UNDERSTANDING THE THREE MASTER
HORMONES   13
Understanding Hormonal Changes in
Perimenopause   13
Hormonal Changes in Menopause   16
The Role of Insulin   17
Cortisol: The Stress Hormone   22
Oxytocin's Influence   27
Understanding Bioidentical Hormones   28
Welcome to the Menopause Management Quiz   30

2. EXPLORING THE MENOPAUSAL
SYMPHONY OF SYMPTOMS   39
Understanding Insomnia during Menopause   40
Tackling Hot Flashes   45
Managing Mood Swings   52
Addressing Weight Gain   53
Chapter 2 Menopause Management Quiz:
Managing Mood Swings   56

3. LIVING WELL—DIET AND NUTRITION IN
MENOPAUSE   63
Nutritional Needs during Menopause   64
Managing Weight with Diet   70
Supplements for Menopausal Support   74
The Role of Phytoestrogens   76
Chapter 3 Menopause Management Quiz:
Unlocking Your Inner Chef   78

4. LEAPING FORWARD—PHYSICAL ACTIVITY
AND EXERCISE FOR MENOPAUSE   87
Exercise for Hormonal Balance   87
Cardiovascular Exercise   89
Strength Training and Bone Health   91
Flexibility and Balance Exercises   93
Chapter 4 Menopause Management Quiz: Find
Your Inner Wellness Warrior   95

5. NURTURING HEALTH—HOLISTIC AND
ALTERNATIVE THERAPIES   103
Herbal and Natural Remedies   103
Best Herbal Teas   105
Body Therapies   106
Energy Healing Techniques   109
Cultivating a Healthy Microbiome for Menopause   113
Chapter 5 Menopause Management Quiz:
Unlocking Your Inner Herbalist   118

6. EMBRACING COMMUNITY—BUILDING A
SUPPORT NETWORK FOR MENOPAUSE   125
Recognizing the Importance of Support   125
Nurturing Family and Friendships   127
Professional Support and Counseling   134
Leveraging Technology for Support   137
Chapter 6 Menopause Management Quiz:
Unlocking Your Support Squad   141

7. STAYING BALANCED—MENOPAUSE AND
MENTAL WELL-BEING   145
Recognizing Signs of Depression   145
Anxiety in Menopause   147
Cognitive Function and Brain Health   149
Self-Care and Relaxation   153
Building Resilience and Empowerment   157
Chapter 7 Menopause Management Quiz:
Nurturing Your Mind & Body   159

8. STEPPING INTO THE FUTURE—
   NAVIGATING POST-MENOPAUSE   165
   Future Focused Health: Beyond Menopause   165
   Embracing New Horizons   170
   Advancing Personal Development   173
   Global Perspectives on Post-Menopause   176
   Chapter 8 Menopause Management Quiz: A
   Guide to Post-Menopausal Empowerment   181

   Conclusion   185
   References   189

Medical Disclaimer:

The information provided in this book is for general informational purposes only and is not intended to be a substitute for professional medical advice, diagnosis, or treatment. Always seek the advice of your physician or other qualified healthcare provider with any questions you may have regarding a medical condition. Never disregard professional medical advice or delay seeking it because of something you have read in this book

Trigger Warning: This book contains discussions and descriptions of menopausal symptoms and related experiences, which may be triggering or distressing for some readers. Menopause is a natural biological process that can involve physical, emotional, and psychological changes, and the content of this book may include detailed accounts of these experiences.

Some topics covered in this book may include hot flashes, mood swings, changes in libido, sleep disturbances, and other symptoms commonly associated with menopause. Additionally, there may be discussions about the impact of menopause on relationships, self-esteem, and overall well-being.

If you are currently experiencing or have a history of mental health challenges, trauma, or sensitivity to discussions about bodily changes, we advise proceeding with caution while reading this book. It's important to prioritize your emotional well-being and seek support from a qualified healthcare professional or counselor if needed.

Introduction

The world of menopause is a scientific and medical wonder. Did you know that most women are often confused about when we are in menopause or how long it lasts? Menopause typically occurs naturally between the ages of 45 and 55. During the transition phase known as "perimenopause," menstrual periods become irregular and start to decrease. Once a woman has gone 12 months in a row without a period, she is considered to have reached menopause. But guess what; if you have a period, after, say, six months, that clock starts all over again. Now brace yourself; it typically lasts seven years but can last as long as 14 years (*What Is Menopause?* 2021).

Meet Christine, the perpetual youngest among her friend group, a fact she never hesitated to remind everyone. As her companions embarked on their menopausal odyssey, previously delicately referred to as "The Change," Christine remained blissfully ignorant. She would show up for girls' weekends with her flannel pajamas, fuzzy slippers, and extra blankets and see the chagrined expression on their faces. "We would suffocate in our sleep if we wore all that," they'd say with a rueful laugh.

Early the next morning, she walked into the bathroom and watched as her best friend plucked a dark chin hair with a pair of tweezers. "Oh, you need a great magnifying mirror, hon; it makes such a difference when you're taming these stray eyebrow hairs."

She shook her head, slightly amused, unaware of what the world of menopause had in store for her.

Not too long after, as she sat in an important meeting one frosty December afternoon, she found herself sweating profusely, her once pristine silk blouse now displaying unsightly perspiration stains, her hair matted to her face. She powered through that meeting, fanning herself with anything close at hands. The minute she got back into her office, she conference-called her good friends. In unison, she heard their voices say, "Welcome to menopause, Christine!"

Christine's tale is familiar to many of us. One moment, we're cruising through life; the next, we're caught in the throes of "power surges"—as I like to call those surprise hot flashes as well as insomnia, mood swings, and that perpetually unwelcome guest —weight gain. It's a journey that can leave us feeling like passengers on a rollercoaster without a seatbelt, our bodies seeming to betray us at every turn.

You're now holding a guidebook crafted especially for modern women like you, navigating the unpredictable terrain of menopause with a mix of wisdom, humor, and practical advice.

Within these pages, you'll find not just medical insights but relatable anecdotes, easy lifestyle adjustments, and holistic therapies designed to help you not just survive but thrive during menopause. I will introduce you to the WELLNESS framework

—a roadmap to reclaiming control over your body and your life.

- **W**isdom in Menopause: Understanding the Three Master Hormones
- **E**xploring the Menopausal Symphony of Symptoms
- **L**iving Well: Diet and Nutrition in Menopause
- **L**eaping Forward: Physical Activity and Exercise for Menopause
- **N**urturing Health: Holistic and Alternative Therapies
- **E**mbracing Community: Building a Support Network for Menopause
- **S**taying Balanced: Menopause and Mental Well-Being
- **S**tepping into the Future: Navigating Post-Menopause

I understand the struggles you face—the sudden surges of heat accompanied by profuse sweating at random and inconvenient times, the emotional upheaval, the sleepless nights spent tossing and turning, and the frustration of jeans that suddenly feel two sizes too small. The goal is to guide you through it all, offering shortcuts to understanding hormonal shifts, simple holistic strategies for symptom relief, and tips for maintaining your sanity and sense of humor along the way.

By the time you reach the end of this journey, you'll emerge not just wiser but stronger and more empowered than ever before. Imagine a life where menopausal symptoms are managed effectively, where you feel balanced, confident, and able to find laughter amidst the chaos and as a bonus you come out on the other side energized and No More Periods!

Gone are the days of navigating menopause alone, armed with nothing but a handful of outdated advice or uncomfortable silence. With this comprehensive guide, you'll be equipped with the knowledge and tools you need to tackle menopause head-on, armed with a modern, renewed sense of vitality.

So, take a deep breath, and let's embark on this journey. Menopause may be a ride filled with unexpected twists and turns, but with the right guidance, it can also be a thrilling adventure— one that leads to a future filled with health, happiness, and endless possibilities.

Chapter 1

Wisdom in Menopause—Understanding the Three Master Hormones

I magine your hormones as members of a seasoned jazz band. For years, they've played in perfect sync, creating a rhythm that's kept everything from your energy to your moods in tune. But here comes menopause, stepping in like an impromptu solo, throwing off the band's groove. In this chapter, we'll get up close and personal with our lead players—estrogen, progesterone, and testosterone—to understand their new solos in the menopause jazz club. Get ready for some insightful notes and a few humorous beats as we learn how to swing to the rhythm of menopause.

Understanding Hormonal Changes in Perimenopause

So, what exactly is perimenopause? Think of it as your body's way of saying, "Hey, I'm getting ready for menopause!" During this time, your ovaries start producing less hormones, especially estrogen, leading to some pretty funky changes in your menstrual cycle. It's like your body's own version of a disco party—unpredictable and full of surprises. According to MyAlloy.com, 6,000 women reach menopause in the U.S. every day, and 80% of them report a wide variety of symptoms.

Estrogen

As the superstar of female hormones, estrogen plays a crucial role in maintaining the health and well-being of the female reproductive system. Often likened to a fairy godmother, estrogen ensures that everything stays healthy, happy, and well-hydrated "down there." However, during perimenopause, estrogen levels can become unpredictable, leading to a game of hide-and-seek within our bodies. (*Perimenopause*, 2021).

Progesterone and Testosterone

During perimenopause, the levels of progesterone and even a touch of testosterone are doing the cha-cha. At the same time, while the sporadic dips in progesterone can throw menstrual cycles for a loop, the age-related decline in testosterone might just put a damper on libido (*Perimenopause*, 2021). Ah, the joys of hormonal shenanigans.

Now, don't be alarmed if perimenopause crashes your party anytime between your mid-30s to mid-50s. It's a bit like being stuck in traffic—some get through it quickly, while others feel like they're parked there for ages; typically around four to eight years (Mayo Clinic Staff, 2023).

During this hormonal rodeo, your body might throw in some extra fun like:

- irregular periods
- mood swings
- vaginal dryness

- hot flashes
- breast tenderness
- insomnia
- weight gain
- headaches
- low sex drive
- depression
- fatigue
- night sweats
- brain fog
- heart palpitations
- thinning hair
- facial hair

(Mayo Clinic Staff, 2023)

It's your body's way of saying, "Hey, let's shake things up a bit!"

But fear not, my fellow goddesses—you're not alone in this adventure. We're all in the same boat, navigating the twists and turns of perimenopause together.

And guess what? You can still get pregnant during this time. So, if you're not ready to hang up your baby-making boots, you might want to keep that in mind. Has anybody ever heard of that "change of life baby"? An unexpected bundle of joy just when you thought production had shut down.

When does the wild ride part come to an end? Well, once you've gone a full 12 continuous months without Aunt Flo paying a visit, congratulations—you've officially reached menopause. Cue the confetti and celebration music.

Hormonal Changes in Menopause

Picture your body as a thriving garden, with estrogen and progesterone as your skilled gardeners nurturing the delicate balance of growth and tranquility. During perimenopause, these two hormones are experts, sometimes working together and other times spinning off on their own unpredictable paths. But when menopause hits, the plan changes. Estrogen takes a sudden dive, triggering those familiar weeds like hot flashes, sleep disruptions, and mood swings to sprout up front and center. Meanwhile, testosterone, the hormone that fuels your passion and vitality, decides to take a vacation, leaving you feeling a tad less vibrant. The garden begins to feel overwhelming.

Now, here's where things get really interesting. Your thyroid, the little gland in your neck with a big job, decides to join the party, too. It's like that friend who always shows up uninvited but ends up playing a crucial role. At this stage, the risk of your thyroid going a bit wonky increases, and it loves to mimic those pesky menopausal symptoms like fatigue and weight gain. Talk about a double whammy, so be aware.

It's estimated that up to 20% of women over 60 might be dealing with a sluggish thyroid alongside menopause (Mukherjee, 2023). These symptoms love to mirror menopause just to keep you on your toes. It is important to discuss all your symptoms with your healthcare team and rule out health concerns. We don't want to "assume" all our symptoms are just menopause.

Together, you can untangle the web of symptoms and come up with a game plan. Whether it's tweaking your hormone levels or giving your thyroid a little extra TLC, there are plenty of options to help you feel like yourself again.

The Role of Insulin

Here's the scoop: low blood sugar can trigger those fiery hot flashes, while on the flip side, experiencing worse hot flashes could be linked to higher blood sugars. It's a blood sugar seesaw, and that can play havoc with multiple symptoms.

First off, let's talk about blood sugar management. Tempting as it may be to drown your sorrows in a mountain of sugary treats, resist the urge. Instead, opt for slow-release sugars with a low glycemic index (GI) food. My favorite is a sweet flavorful nectarine. Some examples are:

- **Non-starchy vegetables**: Think leafy greens like spinach, kale, and Swiss chard, as well as cruciferous veggies like broccoli, cauliflower, asparagus, and Brussels sprouts. These fiber-rich wonders are like nature's broomsticks, sweeping away any blood sugar spikes.
- **Whole grains**: Opt for grains like organic barley, bulgur, and old-fashioned oats. These complex carbs are like the marathon runners of the food world, providing sustained energy without the crash and burn.
- **Nuts and seeds**: Chia seeds, walnuts, almonds, and flaxseeds are your go-to. These crunchy delights are not only tasty but also loaded with healthy fats and protein, keeping your blood sugar levels in check.
- **Berries**: The number one healthiest fruits are blueberries, followed by strawberries, raspberries, and blackberries—all low in sugar but high in flavor and fiber. They're like little flavor bombs that won't send your blood sugar on a rollercoaster ride.
- **Yogurt**: Opt for plain Greek yogurt, which is rich in protein and low in added sugars. It's like a creamy, tangy

superhero that keeps your blood sugar levels steady with the added benefit of keeping your gut happy.

- **Sweet potatoes**: Swap out regular white potatoes for organic sweet potatoes (no, yams are not the same thing), which are packed with vitamins, minerals, and fiber. They're the sweet-tasting, nutritious cousins of the spud family, providing slow-burning energy without the sugar rush (Mayo Clinic Staff, 2022).

If you're already juggling diabetes along with menopause, don't panic. Just keep tabs on those blood sugars and stay in contact with your doctor. Knowledge is power, my friends, and a little sugar monitoring can go a long way (Mayo Clinic Staff, 2022).

Insulin Resistance and Menopause

Picture insulin as the big shot in the hormone world, with its fingers in many pies—including diabetes, obesity, heart disease, and polycystic ovarian syndrome (PCOS). It's like the conductor of a symphony, and when it's out of tune, the whole orchestra (a.k.a. your body) starts playing the wrong notes.

Here's the kicker: during menopause, your body's already juggling a hormonal circus, trying to keep up with fluctuating levels of estrogen, progesterone, and testosterone. Now, add insulin resistance to the mix, and it's like throwing a monkey wrench into already chaotic machinery.

You see, when insulin isn't playing nice, it messes with your other hormones, leaving you feeling like you're stuck in a hormonal avalanche with no end in sight. Hot flashes, weight gain, fatigue —you name it, insulin resistance can make it worse.

Your diet plays a starring role in this drama. Eating too many simple carbs, like white or brown sugar, white rice, white pasta, regular soda, honey, molasses, and most syrups (especially the dreaded high-fructose corn syrup), fuels the fire of insulin resistance. It's like giving a toddler a tub of candy—chaos ensues.

But fear not, we're not doomed to suffer the wrath of insulin resistance forever. By making smart choices—think balanced meals and regular exercise—you can kick insulin resistance to the curb and reclaim your vitality.

Diet's Impact on Insulin

What we eat has a big impact on our insulin levels. Think of it like this—certain foods can cause our insulin levels to spike, while others help keep them steady.

To keep that insulin balanced and happy, aim for a diet that's like a colorful rainbow on your plate. Load up on lean meats and proteins (think chicken, fish, tofu), toss in some high-fiber grains (like oats, barley, millet, buckwheat, and farro), and don't forget to pile on those veggies and legumes. Leafy greens and fruit are your pals, too, so let them join the party.

Now, if you're already dealing with the issue of insulin resistance, here's a game plan to tackle it head-on:

- **Mind those carbs:** When it comes to managing your carb intake during menopause, quality matters. Opt for nutrient-rich sources like vegetables and fruits, which provide essential vitamins, minerals, and fiber without the added sugars and refined grains found in bread and pasta. Aim for around 15 grams of carbohydrates per meal, paired with lean protein, to promote satiety and stabilize blood sugar levels. For snacks, keep it light with approximately seven grams of similar carbs to keep cravings at bay and maintain steady energy levels throughout the day.

- **Embrace healthy fats:** Essential fatty acids (EFAs) play a crucial role in hormone regulation and overall health, making them a vital component of your menopausal diet. Incorporate sources of healthy fats such as avocados, cold-water fish like salmon, flax seeds, and eggs into your meals to support hormone balance and promote heart health. If you're not able to get enough EFAs from food alone, consider adding an omega-3 supplement to ensure you're meeting your body's needs.

- **Supercharge with supplements:** The fact that menopause can throw your hormones for a loop, leading to pesky carb and sugar cravings, can derail your wellness efforts when dealing with insulin resistance or diabetes. Consider complementing your diet with a complete nutritional supplement specially formulated to support hormonal balance and curb cravings. These supplements can provide essential nutrients and botanical extracts that may be lacking in your diet, helping you navigate the ups and downs of perimenopause and menopause with greater ease and resilience.

- **Chill out:** Stress is not just a mental burden—it can also have profound effects on your physical health, including insulin resistance and blood sugar dysregulation. Make stress management a priority in your menopausal wellness routine by incorporating relaxation techniques such as yoga, meditation, deep breathing exercises, or simply indulging in activities that bring you joy and peace. By taking time to unwind and recharge, you'll not only support your hormonal balance but also enhance your overall well-being and vitality.

- **Lifestyle tweaks:** As you navigate the menopausal transition, making small but impactful lifestyle changes can make a world of difference in managing your blood chemistry and supporting your overall health. Quitting smoking, moderating alcohol intake, and prioritizing quality sleep are all key components of a healthy lifestyle during menopause. By ditching unhealthy habits and embracing self-care practices, you'll lay the foundation for a vibrant and fulfilling life beyond menopause.

By incorporating these strategies into your daily routine, you'll not only navigate the challenges of menopause with greater ease and resilience but also emerge stronger, healthier, and more empowered than ever before. So, let's embrace these tools and techniques as we embark on this transformative journey together, supporting each other every step of the way.

Exercise and Insulin Sensitivity

Insulin resistance basically means your body's cells aren't responding to insulin like they need to, leading to higher blood sugar levels. It's a pretty common phenomenon during menopause. According to some studies, about 30–40% of post-menopausal women experience insulin resistance (Matsui et al., 2013).

Regular physical activity is like a secret weapon against insulin resistance. When you get moving, whether it's some yoga stretches, a brisk walk, or even a dance session in your living room, you're telling your cells to perk up and pay attention to insulin again. Studies have shown that exercise can improve insulin sensitivity, helping to keep those blood sugar levels in check (Stills, 2013).

Plus, let's not forget the other perks of exercise during menopause. It's like a natural mood booster, waving away mood swings and giving you a dose of those feel-good endorphins. And don't even get me started on the benefits for your bone health. With osteoporosis peeking around the corner, even moderate strengthening exercise can help keep your bones strong and sturdy.

Now, I know what you might be thinking: "But I'm not exactly an Olympic athlete here." And hey, that's totally okay. You don't need to be breaking records or bench-pressing your body weight. Regularly engaging in just 30 minutes of moderate exercise most days of the week can have remarkable effects.

So, whether you're dusting off those running shoes, busting out some Zumba moves, or simply taking the dog for a stroll, every little bit counts. Find something you enjoy, and show insulin resistance who's boss.

Cortisol: The Stress Hormone

When you're driving, and suddenly an animal appears in your lane, you can thank cortisol for the rush of energy you get as you try to avoid an accident. If you've experienced a frightening situation like this, that's the hormone that accounts for it.

Cortisol is often referred to as "the stress hormone" because it triggers the fight or flight response. This means it rapidly raises your blood sugar to provide quick energy and also boosts your blood pressure. These effects can be beneficial in life-threatening situations. However, cortisol also reacts to non-life-threatening stressors, such as work deadlines or being stuck in traffic (Johnson, 2020).

Symptoms of high cortisol may include: irritability, headaches, and gastro-intestinal problems like bloating, constipation or diarrhea.

However unpredictable it may be, cortisol continues to play a crucial role in your daily life. For instance, your body typically has elevated cortisol levels upon waking up and during exercise, as this hormone can provide energy and regulate blood pressure. The issues arise from the fact that many individuals have higher-than-normal cortisol levels, with women tending to have higher levels than men. This can lead to various bodily issues, including symptoms similar to those experienced during menopause, such as:

- fatigue
- brain fog
- anxiety
- depression
- increased belly fat
- mood swings

Kathy's Story

Kathy knows this struggle all too well. She's the poster child for healthy living, yet her "menopause muffin top" was growing faster than flowers in springtime.

For a whole year, Kathy tried everything under the sun: changing her diet, cutting back on wine, ramping up those evening walks, but nothing seemed to affect that stubborn weight gain. Sound familiar? It wasn't until she stumbled upon the cortisol connection that things finally clicked. With her parents needing care, stress had become her constant companion, and her body was hoarding those extra pounds like they were gold.

Armed with newfound knowledge, Kathy decided to wage war on stress with relaxation and stress-reduction techniques. She dabbled in yoga, embraced meditation like it was a long-lost BFF, and made self-care a non-negotiable part of her daily routine.

And guess what? The pounds started to melt away like snow in July. Suddenly, that "menopause muffin top" was looking more like a petite cupcake. Kathy's story isn't just about shedding weight; it's about reclaiming control over her health and well-being.

So, what can you do during menopause to help reduce stress and lower high cortisol levels? Making small changes, such as maintaining a balanced diet and engaging in regular exercise three to five days a week, can aid in lowering cortisol levels. Additionally, practicing stress-reduction techniques can improve your well-being and promote relaxation, thereby reducing cortisol and stress responses during menopause.

Here are a few things to consider:

- **Identify the sources of your stress.** Understanding the root causes of your stress is the first step toward effective management. Take some time to reflect on the specific situations, tasks, or activities that are contributing to your stress levels. Is there a particular aspect of your work or personal life that feels overwhelming? Are there relationship dynamics that could be improved? Once you've identified these stressors, brainstorm alternative approaches or solutions that could help alleviate their impact. Don't hesitate to reach out for support from friends, family, or professional resources if needed. Sometimes, simply talking through your concerns with someone you trust can provide valuable perspective and relief.

- **Remember to prioritize your physical well-being.** Menopause symptoms can take a toll on your physical health, exacerbating feelings of stress and being overwhelmed. It's essential to prioritize self-care and seek guidance from your doctor if you're struggling with severe symptoms. Your healthcare provider can offer personalized advice and explore treatment options tailored to your needs, whether it's hormone therapy, dietary changes, or alternative therapies. By addressing your physical well-being, you'll be better equipped to cope with the demands of daily life and manage stress more effectively.

- **Consider making positive lifestyle changes.** The way you feed and move your body can significantly impact your stress levels and overall well-being. Embrace a balanced and nourishing diet rich in fruits, vegetables, whole grains, and lean proteins to fuel your body and support optimal health. Regular physical activity, such as walking, swimming, or yoga, can also help reduce stress and boost your mood by releasing endorphins, the body's natural stress reliever. Additionally, reducing or steering clear of stimulants like caffeine, alcohol, and nicotine can promote better sleep and overall well-being, making it easier to manage stress effectively.

- **Consider practicing mindfulness to help alleviate stress.** Mindfulness techniques, such as meditation, yoga, or Tai Chi, can be powerful tools for reducing stress and promoting relaxation. These practices encourage you to focus on the present moment and cultivate a sense of calm and inner peace. Whether you carve out a few minutes each day for meditation or attend a yoga class to unwind, incorporating mindfulness into your routine can help soothe your mind and body amidst the chaos of daily life. Engaging in fulfilling hobbies or activities that bring you joy and fulfillment can also serve as a form of mindfulness, allowing you to immerse yourself fully in the present moment and escape from stressors temporarily.

- **Counseling or talk therapies can also provide support.** If you find yourself struggling to cope with stress despite your best efforts, don't hesitate to seek professional support. Counseling or talk therapies, such as cognitive-behavioral therapy (CBT), can provide you with valuable tools and strategies for managing stress more effectively. Through CBT, you'll learn to identify and challenge negative thought patterns and develop healthier coping mechanisms for dealing with stressors. A trained therapist can offer guidance, support, and encouragement as you work toward greater resilience and well-being.

By implementing these stress management strategies into your daily life, you'll empower yourself to navigate the challenges of menopause with greater ease and resilience. Remember, managing stress is a journey, and it's okay to seek support and guidance along the way. With a proactive approach to self-care and stress management, you'll cultivate a greater sense of balance, peace, and well-being in your life.

But you should also be aware; not only are we negatively affected by high cortisol levels, we can also experience low cortisol. You might need to check in with your doctor if you are constantly fatigued and have difficulty focusing, or have sugar and salt cravings.

Oxytocin's Influence

Let's talk about one of the good hormones we need to promote during menopause: oxytocin. Yep, that's right, the same cuddle hormone that makes you feel all warm and fuzzy when hugging loved ones. This hormone is a powerhouse player in your menopausal journey.

First up, let's talk about bonding and emotional wellness. That menopause roller coaster can get out of hand through a maze of emotions, right? Well, oxytocin swoops in like a caped crusader, promoting feelings of trust, love, and connection. So, next time you're feeling a bit wobbly emotionally, call up a friend, hug your pet, or schedule a Zoom chat with your favorite people. It's like a mini oxytocin boost.

Now, onto the steamy stuff: oxytocin and sexual health. Menopause might throw a few curveballs your way in the bedroom department. Oxytocin can come to the rescue once again. It's been dubbed the "love hormone" for a reason—it can enhance intimacy, arousal, and even orgasm. So, don't be shy about getting cozy with your partner or exploring solo adventures. Your body has more tricks up its sleeve than you might think.

You can enhance oxytocin naturally. Yep, you heard me right. Exercise, meditation, massage, laughter—all of these can give your oxytocin levels a nudge in the right direction. So, make time for activities that make you feel good inside and out. Your body and mind will thank you for it.

Now, let's talk about mood regulation. Ah, the challenges of mood swings during menopause. Oxytocin steps in as your trusty sidekick here, helping to keep those mood swings in check. It's like having your own personal mood stabilizer, working behind the scenes to keep you feeling balanced and grounded. So, when you have one of those days when everything seems to irritate you, engage in "operation oxytocin dump," as I like to call it. Get a massage, hug someone, try yoga, listen to music or make some music of your own, spend time with friends, and meditate on the good things in your life. Watch a few cat videos on YouTube. Do any activity that brings you joy or laughter. Allow your body to be flooded with that happy hormone and turn that frown upside down (Santos, 2018).

Understanding Bioidentical Hormones

What are bioidentical hormones? Well, think of them as nature's little helpers. Bioidentical hormones are derived from plant sources, like yams or soy, and they mimic the hormones your body naturally produces (*Bioidentical Hormones*, 2022). Yep, they're like the VIP pass to hormone harmony.

When it comes to managing menopause, bioidentical hormones can be a total game-changer. They can help alleviate those ever-present hot flashes, mood swings, and sleep disturbances. Plus, they're tailored to your unique hormonal needs, making them a personalized solution for your menopausal journey.

Before you go diving headfirst into the bioidentical hormone pool, it's crucial to consult with healthcare professionals. These are the professionals with the medical know-how to help you navigate the ins and outs of hormone therapy.

Consulting with healthcare pros isn't just about getting the green light for hormone therapy; it's also about creating a whole-body approach to your menopause management. They can help you explore other lifestyle changes, like diet, exercise, and stress management techniques, that can complement hormone therapy and boost overall well-being. It's a concerted effort... get it?

Who Shouldn't Take Them

Using hormone therapy involves making a decision with your healthcare provider after considering the risks and benefits. Bioidentical hormones have been controversial, and many are not FDA-approved, but your healthcare provider may still consider them a desirable treatment option. The term Hormone Replacement Therapy or HRT is now referred to as Menopausal Hormone Treatment or MHT. Just be aware that MHT is not intended to replace your hormones at the levels they were prior to menopause. The goal is simply to use the amount of hormone that adequately treats menopausal symptoms. The amount of estrogen used with MHT is much less than the ovaries normally produce at ovulation and at least one-half to one-third the amount of estrogen in a low-dose oral contraceptive. Though MHT is considered safe and effective for the majority of healthy menopausal women, it is important to speak to a doctor about the right treatment for you.

If you have experienced or are at high risk for the following conditions, hormone therapy may not be safe:

- breast cancer
- blood clotting disorders
- stroke
- heart or cardiovascular disease

(*Bioidentical Hormones*, 2022)

Remember, sisterhood is powerful, and you're not alone in this journey. So, lean on your healthcare team, surround yourself with supportive friends and family, and embrace this phase of life with optimism and enthusiasm.

Understanding the three master hormones in menopause marks an essential starting point on your journey. However, it's merely scratching the surface of this transformative phase. As we dive deeper into Chapter 2, we'll unravel the complexities beyond hormones. Menopause isn't just about estrogen, progesterone, and testosterone—it's a multifaceted symphony of symptoms we'll navigate together, exploring the causes, effects, and effective management strategies. Chapter 2 is an enlightening ride through the diverse range of menopausal symptoms, but first, take a short quiz to fix in your mind the points you need to work on to improve your quality of life through your menopause journey.

Welcome to the Menopause Management Quiz

This quiz is designed to help you assess your current strategies for managing menopause symptoms and discover areas where you can focus on a more harmonious experience. So, grab your imaginary maracas and get ready to shimmy through some thought-provoking questions.

Remember, there are no right or wrong answers. Be honest with yourself, and most importantly, have fun!

Instructions: For each statement, choose the response that best reflects your current habits or experiences.

Diet:

1. I prioritize fruits, vegetables, and whole grains in my meals.

- o Often
- o Sometimes
- o Rarely

2. I limit sugary drinks and processed foods.

- o Often
- o Sometimes
- o Rarely

3. I incorporate healthy fats like avocado and nuts into my diet.

- o Often
- o Sometimes
- o Rarely

4. I manage my cravings for sweets and unhealthy snacks.

- o Often
- o Sometimes
- o Rarely

Exercise:

1. I engage in at least 30 minutes of moderate-intensity exercise four to five days a week.

- o Often
- o Sometimes
- o Rarely

2. I find physical activity enjoyable, and it helps me manage stress.

- o Often
- o Sometimes
- o Rarely

3. I prioritize getting enough quality sleep to support my energy levels.

- o Often
- o Sometimes
- o Rarely

4. I make an effort to find time and motivation to exercise regularly.

- o Often
- o Sometimes
- o Rarely

Stress Management:

1. I regularly practice relaxation techniques like yoga or meditation.

- ○ Often
- ○ Sometimes
- ○ Rarely

2. I prioritize activities that bring me joy and reduce stress.

- ○ Often
- ○ Sometimes
- ○ Rarely

3. I make an effort to manage stress and its impact on my well-being.

- ○ Often
- ○ Sometimes
- ○ Rarely

4. I explore different stress management techniques.

- ○ Often
- ○ Sometimes
- ○ Rarely

Understanding Hormones:

1. I am aware of the different hormones involved in menopause and their effects.

- ○ Often
- ○ Sometimes
- ○ Rarely

2. I track my symptoms and can identify potential triggers.

- ○ Often
- ○ Sometimes
- ○ Rarely

3. I feel empowered to make informed decisions about my health during menopause.

- ○ Often
- ○ Sometimes
- ○ Rarely

4. I am happy to discuss my menopause symptoms with health-care professionals.

- ○ Often
- ○ Sometimes
- ○ Rarely

5. What is my current understanding of bioidentical hormones?

- ○ I know very little about them.
- ○ I have heard some basic information but would like to learn more.
- ○ I have researched them and have a good understanding of their potential benefits and risks.

Your Results:

Based on your responses, you might want to focus on the following areas:

- **Diet:** If you answered "rarely" for questions about healthy eating habits, consider exploring resources and recipes for menopause-friendly meals. Learn more about the Mediterranean diet and avoid inflammatory foods like "The Whites" (white sugar, white flour, white potatoes, white rice).
- **Exercise:** If you answered "rarely" for questions about physical activity, start small and find enjoyable ways to move your body. Try a YouTube video for 20 minutes of gentle Tai Chi, or learn a kicky country line dance for fun movements.
- **Stress Management:** If you answered "rarely" for questions about feeling overwhelmed by stress, explore relaxation techniques and prioritize activities you enjoy. Give yourself permission to take a deep breath and center yourself as you determine the next steps in your life journey. And remember, don't sweat the small stuff… and it's all small stuff.
- **Understanding Hormones:** If you answered "rarely" for questions about hormone knowledge,

explore reliable sources of information and consult with healthcare professionals. Additionally, if you are interested in bioidentical hormones, make sure to have a comprehensive discussion with your healthcare provider to understand the potential benefits and risks in your specific case.

Remember, this is just a starting point. Celebrate your strengths and identify areas for growth as you continue your menopause journey.

Disclaimer: This quiz is intended for informational purposes only and does not constitute medical advice. Please consult with your healthcare provider for personalized recommendations.

NOTES:

_____

_____

_____

_____

_____

_____

_____

_____

_____

_____

_____

Chapter 2

Exploring the Menopausal Symphony of Symptoms

You're seated in a grand concert hall, surrounded by a symphony of sounds, each instrument contributing to a masterpiece of music. Now, imagine that each note, every crescendo, and every subtle harmony represents a symptom of menopause. Intriguing, isn't it?

As we embark on this chapter, I invite you to take a seat in the conductor's chair. Let's explore this symphony of symptoms together, understanding each one as if it were a musical instrument in our ensemble. Some symptoms may roar like a trumpet, demanding attention with their boldness—think hot flashes and night sweats, stealing the spotlight when least expected. Others whisper softly in the background, like chin hairs and sleep disturbances, their persistent melody weaving through the fabric of our daily lives.

We're not mere spectators in this performance. No, we are conductors armed with knowledge, wit, and a dash of humor, ready to harmonize this cacophony into a beautiful arrangement of well-being and strength. Throughout this journey, we'll delve into the "whys" behind each symptom, unraveling the mysteries of menopause with the precision of a seasoned musician.

Understanding Insomnia during Menopause

Let's dive into a topic that's probably been haunting your nights lately: insomnia. As if we don't have enough on our plates, we shouldn't have to deal with a lack of sleep to boot. I have some tricks up my sleeve to show insomnia who's boss.

Causes of Menopausal Insomnia

So, why is sleep suddenly playing hard to get? Blame it on the hormonal rollercoaster your body's riding. Estrogen and progesterone, the dynamic duo responsible for regulating your sleep, are throwing a party with their fluctuating levels (*Sleep Problems and Menopause*, 2021). Add in some hot flashes, night sweats, and mood swings, and it's no wonder sleep feels like a distant dream.

Sleep Hygiene Practices

Now, let's talk about getting back in sync with Mr. Sandman. It's time to step up your sleep hygiene game. No, I'm not talking about washing your pillows (though that's not a bad idea). I mean creating a bedtime routine that tells your body, "Hey, it's time to wind down."

Sayonara, screens! Seriously, believe it when I tell you those smartphones and tablets are like sleep's arch-nemesis. The blue light messes with your melatonin production, making it harder to catch those Z's. Ditch the blue light monsters, it's more important now than ever to choose a book instead.

Warm milk, anyone? No, I'm not channeling Grandma here (although she was onto something). A soothing cup of herbal tea can work wonders in calming those pre-bedtime jitters.

Natural Sleep Aids

When the traditional method of counting sheep fails, it may be necessary to seek additional support. This is where natural sleep aids come in. Numerous well-researched and potent supplements for sleep issues can also provide relief from menopausal symptoms, aiding in navigating the menopausal transition with improved well-being, cognition, and performance (Breus, 2018).

Let's discuss some of the most effective supplements for promoting sleep and how they can also help alleviate menopause symptoms. Always talk to your healthcare team before starting any new supplements.

Melatonin

You probably know melatonin as something to help you sleep, but did you know it can also tackle other menopause symptoms? It's not a sedative. Whether your body makes it naturally or you take it as a supplement, melatonin helps your body keep its internal clock in check, making it easier to stick to a regular sleep routine. It can help you fall asleep faster, sleep better overall, and feel less tired during the day. Plus, it might even improve the quality of your sleep and protect your brain and body from cell damage, thanks to its antioxidant superpowers. So melatonin isn't just for sleep—it's amazing for your whole body (Breus, 2018).

Magnolia Bark

Studies have shown that the special compounds in magnolia bark can help you fall asleep faster and spend more time in both deep and dream sleep. Magnolia also calms you down by reducing adrenaline, making it a great natural remedy for those who feel stressed or wired (Breus, 2018).

L-Theanine

Ever heard of L-theanine? It's an amino acid found in tea leaves. This little guy is great at helping you relax, deal with anxiety and mood, and sleep better, but it won't knock you out during the day. L-theanine can help you drift off to sleep faster and improve the quality of your sleep by calming anxiety, not by making you drowsy like a sedative would. So, if you're looking for a natural way to unwind and get some quality shut-eye, L-theanine might just be your new best friend (Breus, 2018).

Magnesium L-threonate

Think of magnesium as a super supplement for sleep and overall health. It helps our body's enzymes work properly, which is key for pretty much everything our body does. It's one of the seven essential minerals we need a lot of, and having enough magnesium keeps our metabolism healthy, mood steady, stress levels low, sleep on track, and hearts and bones strong. It's like a one-stop shop for feeling good inside and out (Breus, 2018).

5-Hydroxytryptophan

A compound our bodies make naturally from the amino acid L-tryptophan, which we get from foods like tuna, chicken, turkey, milk, oats and chocolate. However, as we get older, our natural levels of 5-HTP decrease. Why does 5-HTP matter? Because it helps our bodies produce more serotonin, a neurotransmitter that's like our mood and sleep manager. When serotonin levels are good, we feel happier, sleep better, and our bodies work better overall. Serotonin also helps with digestion, appetite, and how we feel pain. So, keeping our 5-HTP levels up means keeping our serotonin levels up—and that's a win for our mood, sleep, and general well-being (Breus, 2018).

Valerian and Hops

These two supplements are often used together because they're great at improving sleep. They work by boosting GABA, a calming chemical in our brains that helps us relax and sleep better. Lots of studies have shown that valerian, either on its own or with hops, can really help with that all important REM sleep. It helps people fall asleep faster, sleep better overall, and even ease insomnia symptoms. Research specifically focusing on women going through menopause found that valerian is especially helpful for improving sleep. So, if you're struggling to catch those Z's, valerian and hops might be worth a try (Breus, 2018).

Designing a Sleep-Friendly Environment

Alright, let's set the stage for a snooze-worthy slumber. The hot new term is sleep hygiene but your bedroom should be a sanctuary, a haven of relaxation. Designing a bedroom that helps you sleep better is a solid first step toward good sleep hygiene. We need to be mindful of practicality and visual design, lighting, smells and sound levels.

Let's begin with color. The bedding, walls, and accessories should all be a color that evokes calm and rest within you. Your favorite color might be red, but walking into a room that is meant for sleep with stark red walls can conflict with your brain. When choosing, keep asking yourself, "Do these colors make me exhale?"

Regardless of budget or square footage, you want to avoid feeling cramped in your bedroom. Avoid buying a bed that fills the entire space. Think less is more when decorating the walls. Avoid clutter at all costs. Having an open and airy feeling will trick your brain into relaxing and sleeping better.

When you are choosing decor and accessories, look for things that make you smile. You want to enter your bedroom and feel at home. You want that room to welcome you with open arms. Maybe that involves a cozy blanket that reminds you of your grandmother or a framed photo of your children on the dresser. Whatever that looks like for you, do it.

Now, let's be practical.

Lighting is very important for your circadian rhythm. When it gets dark, that is the cue for your brain to shut down and sleep. Black-out curtains work wonders for this. If you keep your windows bare, allowing light pollution in all night, your rhythm will be thrown out of whack (Suni, 2023).

You also need to be mindful of artificial light. A good rule of thumb is to shut down all electronic devices at least one hour before bedtime. Allowing your brain to detox from all that nasty blue light helps it realize it is time to sleep. This includes those of you who have televisions in your bedroom (Suni, 2023).

Have you ever considered the noise level in your bedroom? Maybe you live in an apartment building or close to a fire station. Do you have a noisy roommate or young children? Some of these are out of our control, so you may want to try a white noise machine or earplugs to help. You can also experiment with music apps on your phone that play soothing and relaxing tones, or even the sound of rainfall to promote sleep.

Temperature is the last big one. It is suggested that you should have the temp set between 60 to 71 degrees Fahrenheit, as studies suggest cooler temperatures warrant better sleep (Suni, 2023).

Tackling Hot Flashes

I would like to tell you a story about my friend, we'll call her Michelle. She is in the prime of her life, rocking her career, enjoying her life when menopause catches her completely by surprise. She's never spoken about this with her mother, sisters, or friends. Suddenly, she finds herself dealing with hot flashes so intense she's convinced she could fry an egg on her forehead. Night sweats? More like night swimming competition in her own sheets.

Michelle had no idea how common this was and discovered that approximately three-quarters of women in perimenopause are part of the hot flash club. According to the North American Menopause Society (NAMS), once you hit menopause, those hot flashes might stick around for a while. How long? Let's just say Michelle almost fell over when she realized she could be dealing with these unwanted power surges for anywhere from six months to five years. She even read that in some unlucky cases, you could be stuck with them for a decade or more (Vroomen, 2020).

So, what's a gal to do in the face of such fiery foes? Well, fear not, my fellow warrior queens. I have great tips, tricks, and ice packs just for you.

Hot Flash Triggers

Each woman's personal recipe for triggering hot flashes may vary, but a few popular ingredients include:

- sipping on alcohol
- indulging in caffeinated delights
- savoring spicy treats
- lounging in the heat

- battling stress or anxiety
- rocking snug attire
- puffing on a cigarette
- leaning forward or hunching over

(Vroomen, 2020)

You might consider starting a journal to track your symptoms. Jot down what you were up to, munching on, sipping, feeling, or wearing when each hot flash struck. After a few weeks, you might uncover a pattern that can help you dodge certain triggers.

Dietary Modifications

Battling hot flashes can lead to insomnia and irritability, and what you eat can really shake up how you feel. Here are some top-notch staples to keep in stock:

- **Fruits and vegetables:** Don't forget that rainbow on your plate to beat those hot flashes. Fruits and veggies are like the superheroes of the food world, packed with antioxidants that shield your cells from harm. Think of them as your personal bodyguards, ready to kick those hot flashes to the curb. Get in the habit of reaching for the dark green leafy veggies like spinach, broccoli, and kale. And don't forget about the colorful fruits like cherries, mangoes, and berries; they're like flashy sidekicks, adding some pizzazz to your plate while fighting off those unwanted hot flashes.
- **Fatty fish:** It turns out those omega-3 fatty acids in fish are like superpowers for your mood and brain. They're also secret agents for regulating blood pressure, which means they might just be the hot flash busters we've

been looking for. My favorite lunch is fresh kale salad with dried cranberries, salmon, avocado and a few walnuts in an olive oil and balsamic vinegar dressing.

- **Cooling foods:** It's time to chill out those hot flashes with some "cooling foods" straight from the wisdom of Chinese medicine. Reach for crisp cool apples, spinach, eggs, broccoli, and green tea to turn down the heat. It's like giving your body a frosty treat while packing in delicious nutrients and disease-fighting goodness. So, the next time you're feeling the heat, cool off with these tasty options and let your body thank you with a sigh of relief.

- **Water:** Keep cool and sip on. There's a reason you always hear that you should drink eight glasses, eight ounces each, of pure fresh water daily. Yes, 64 ounces or two liters of water can be the make-it or break-it component of a healthy body. Staying hydrated during menopause is key—give your body a refreshing drink to keep those hot flashes at bay. Plus, it's a win-win: water will also help keep your weight in check and give your body a helping hand in flushing out toxins and soaking up all those vital nutrients. So, drink up and stay fabulous.

(Henry Ford Health Staff, n.d.)

It's important to understand what foods can ease menopause symptoms, but we also need to be mindful of the foods that can make our symptoms worse. Let's review a few:

- **Spicy foods:** Keep things cool and avoid turning up the heat with spicy foods. If you're already feeling the burn from hot flashes or have high blood pressure, it might be time to bid farewell to the jalapeños and cayenne. Trust me, your taste buds will thank you, and you'll avoid feeling like you're breathing fire. So, let's keep it mild and enjoy our meals without the added heat.

- **Alcohol:** Now let's chat about our wine-down time, shall we? Sipping on a 5 ounce glass a few times a week? No biggie. But if you're hitting the bottle like it's happy hour every day, it might be time to rethink your strategy. Alcohol can crash the party by messing with your sleep, cranking up those power surges, and even inviting anxiety and depression to join in on the fun. So, let's raise a glass responsibly and keep the good times flowing without the extra baggage.

(Henry Ford Health Staff, n.d.)

Snacking: Get the munchies late in the evening? Addicted to those late-night raids on the fridge? That might just be the cause of those unwanted pounds crashing your party. Do an experiment for 21 days and see if it could become part of your new healthy routine: No food after 8pm. See if you don't lose those snacking urges, feel less bloated and sleep better, to boot.

Herbal Remedies

Although medical studies have yet to give herbal products a gold star for reducing hot flashes, some women swear by these natural remedies. As always, do your own research and make a note of any patterns of changes, both beneficial and detrimental, when taking supplements.

They include:

- **Black cohosh:** Commonly used for hot flashes, insomnia, and irritability. Try it in a tea; however, it is not recommended if you suffer from a liver disorder.
- **Red clover:** This supplement contains isoflavones, polyphenols, and "phytoestrogens," which are plant-based compounds similar to estrogen. But be aware your chance of bleeding increases if you ingest this.
- **Dong quai**: May reduce inflammation and help to balance hormones. However, if you are prescribed the blood thinner warfarin (Coumadin), you should avoid this herb as it interacts directly with it.
- **Evening primrose oil:** Contains omega-6 fatty acids to help regulate hormone levels, hot flashes, and skin elasticity. Be aware this essential oil can decrease the effectiveness of blood thinners and a few medications used to treat depression and anxiety.
- **Soy:** Contains a variety of phytochemicals and antioxidants and may lower blood pressure and cholesterol levels as well as reduce menopausal symptoms. Do your own research regarding soy. It can cause digestive upset and is not recommended for those who have a history of cancers related to estrogen (Vroomen, 2020).

Always speak with your doctor prior to taking any herbal supplements because they have the potential to interfere with medications, even beyond what is listed here.

How to Cool Down and Be Comfortable

A woman experiencing a hot flash will do anything, and I mean anything, to cool down. Personally, I can be found walking around in the winter in just a T-shirt. I keep a basket of blankets in the living room for others because the windows will remain open all year. Any person who attempts to turn the heat up will be met with the stare of death. So, what can you do to find instant coolness in those moments of intense heat?

- Opt for breezy, lightweight attire.
- Layer up so you can easily shed when you start to sizzle.
- Keep your cool with fans or air conditioning at home, work, or in your ride.
- Keep a nifty handheld fan handy for when you're on the move.
- Stay refreshed with sips of cool water or other chilled beverages.

(Cirino, 2023)

Now, when we are hit with waves of heat during the night, it is a whole new ball game. You can be fast asleep one moment and swimming in your own sweat the next. I know, disgusting. I have a few great suggestions to combat this:

- Steer clear of exercise, caffeine, and alcohol two hours before bedtime.
- Construct a soothing bedtime routine to dial down the stress. Refer to the tips on a calming bedroom and shutting down blue light devices.
- Lower the temperature in your bedroom before hitting the hay.

- Use a ceiling or bedside fan to chill the room while you snooze.
- Opt for lightweight sheets and blankets, and wear loose, airy sleepwear. Bamboo fabric is the best choice to keep moisture away from your body.
- Rotate your pillow during the night to keep the cool side on your face.
- Try a cooling gel pillow or slip an ice pack under your pillow for a refreshing effect.

(Cirino, 2023)

In addition to this, I came up with this great idea after becoming frustrated during my own night sweat escapades. I found myself constantly waking, soaked, and overheated. Not wanting to wake my husband, I would fumble in the dark trying to find dry pajamas, something to drink, and anything to help me cool down.

I now keep what I call "the cooling kit" beside my bed in a small canvas basket. You can use a bag or whatever is convenient for you. Inside, I have the following:

- extra pajamas
- a fresh pillowcase
- extra underwear
- cooling minty wipes (yes, they are a thing)
- an insulated bottle of cold water (refilled each night)
- handheld fan
- two ice packs (they are put in right before bed)

This has made my sweaty wake-up calls just a bit more bearable. I am able to fall back to sleep faster because I spend less time awake trying to find what I need. Give it a try.

Managing Mood Swings

Let's dive into the wild world of mood swings, shall we? Trust me, you're not alone in this rollercoaster ride of emotions. Did you know that about 75% of women experience mood swings during menopause (Villaverde Gutiérrez et al., 2012)?

So, why do these mood swings happen? Well, blame it on the hormonal chaos. As our estrogen levels take a nosedive, it messes with our brain chemistry, leaving us feeling like we're on an emotional seesaw (Villaverde Gutiérrez et al., 2012). One minute, we're laughing; the next, we're crying over a commercial about puppies. Sound familiar?

Did you know that some things we eat can come to our rescue? First up, omega-3 fatty acids. These little darlings found in fish, flaxseeds, and walnuts can help stabilize mood and reduce those mood swings. Then there's magnesium, our chill pill mineral found in spinach, almonds, and dark chocolate. It helps calm the nervous system and keeps mood swings in check (Letts, n.d.).

Now, let's talk about getting our bodies moving. Exercise isn't just about fitting into those skinny jeans (although that's a nice bonus); it's also a powerful mood booster. Whether it's a brisk walk, a yoga session, or a dance party in your living room, getting your heart pumping releases feel-good endorphins that can help combat those mood swings and leave you feeling like yourself again (Villaverde Gutiérrez et al., 2012).

We also need to talk about mindfulness and coping strategies. Picture this: you're feeling like you're about to explode into a ball of emotions. Instead of diving headfirst into a pint of ice cream (although, no judgment if you do), try one of these (Ackerman, 2017):

Body scan meditation:

- Sit or recline in a comfortable position, gently close your eyes, and concentrate on your breathing.
- Scan your body slowly from your toes to your head, observing any tension without judgment.
- Release tension with each breath, fostering relaxation and connection between mind and body.

Gratitude journaling:

- Daily, write three things you're grateful for, big or small.
- Feel gratitude deeply, reflecting on its positive impact, shifting focus from stress to positivity.

Mindful breathing:

- Sit comfortably, close your eyes, and place your hands on your abdomen.
- Inhale deeply through your nose, allowing your belly to expand, then exhale slowly through your mouth, contracting your belly.
- Focus on your breath for several minutes, calming the nervous system and enhancing emotional stability.

Addressing Weight Gain

Studies show that around 90% of women experience some weight gain during menopause, with an average gain of five pounds during the transition phase and up to 15 pounds within a decade post-menopause (*Menopause and Weight*, n.d.). But hey, remember, these numbers aren't destiny; they're just part of the journey. I find it almost mandatory to keep a diet journal. Not only do I keep track of my water intake and the number of grams of protein/carbs/fat I'm eating, but I can also note my feelings after a meal. Bloated? Skip the beans next time. Irritable? Oops, those pesky whites have slipped in. Avoiding white sugar, white flour, white potatoes, and white rice helps in many different ways.

The Metabolic Shift: Understanding What's Going On

Now, let's demystify this metabolic shift. It's like your body decides to shake things up just when you thought you had the game all figured out. As we age, our metabolism naturally slows down, and during menopause, hormonal changes can make it even more sluggish. Estrogen levels drop, messing with our body's fat distribution, while progesterone levels dip, making us prone to storing fat around our midsection (oh joy) (*Menopause and Weight*, n.d.).

Diet Adjustments: Nourish Your Body, Mind, and Spirit

So, what's a savvy sister to do? Time to give your diet a makeover. Think of it as a love letter to your body—water, water, water is mandatory, plus fill up with nutrient-rich foods that keep you feeling energized and satisfied. Concentrate on consuming whole foods such as fruits, vegetables, lean proteins, and healthy fats. Oh, and don't forget the calcium-rich foods to keep those bones strong—your future self will thank you (Bartosch, 2023).

Regular Exercise: Shake What Your Mama Gave Ya!

Alright, let's talk exercise, again. I know, I know, it's not always everyone's cup of tea, but hear me out. Don't let the bathroom scale rule your life because the fact is, muscle weighs more than an equal amount of fat but it takes up less space and burns calories continuously. How great is that? Regular exercise is like hitting the reset button on your metabolism. It helps you burn calories, build muscle (adios, yucky fat), and boost those feel-good endorphins. Plus, it's a fantastic stress-buster—a win-win in my book (Bartosch, 2023).

Managing Cravings and Portion Control: Size Matters

Now, let's tackle those cravings and portion control. Look, we all have that inner snack monster whispering sweet temptations in our ears, but don't let it run the show. Instead, get crafty with your snacks—opt for healthier choices like nuts, Greek yogurt (no added sugar), or a piece of dark chocolate. And when it comes to portions, size matters but portion control isn't about deprivation; it's about savoring every delicious bite without overdoing it (Bartosch, 2023). Ditch the highly processed fatty snack foods full of sugar, salt and chemicals. If it comes in a bag or box, has more than 4 ingredients or has any ingredient you can't pronounce, that my dear, is the opposite of what your body needs.

As we draw the curtain on this chapter discussing the wild and wonderful world of menopausal symptoms, let me first offer you a round of applause. You've made it through some intense hormonal acrobatics, navigating mood swings like a pro and facing hot flashes head-on (pun intended).

As you turn the page, get ready to learn more about how diet and nutrition affect women going through menopause. We will discuss how making informed dietary choices can be a key strategy for living well. I will provide practical dietary guidelines and tailored nutritional advice for menopausal women and explain how these choices can positively impact overall well-being and symptom management during menopause.

Chapter 2 Menopause Management Quiz: Managing Mood Swings

Welcome back, conductors! Now that you've explored the emotional rollercoaster of menopause and learned strategies to manage mood swings prepare to conduct your knowledge like a baton. This quiz will help you understand your own emotional landscape and empower you to navigate it with grace.

Remember, there are no wrong answers. Be honest with yourself, and most importantly, embrace the journey.

Instructions: For each statement, choose the response that best reflects your experience with mood swings during menopause.

Emotional Awareness:

1. I understand what is behind mood swings that disrupt my daily life.

- Often
- Sometimes
- Rarely

2. I am aware of my triggers and situations that worsen my mood swings.

- Often
- Sometimes
- Rarely

3. I recognize the physical sensations associated with my changing moods.

- o Often
- o Sometimes
- o Rarely

4. I explore different strategies to manage my mood swings.

- o Often
- o Sometimes
- o Rarely

Dietary Modifications:

1. I incorporate omega-3 fatty acids and magnesium into my diet.

- o Often
- o Sometimes
- o Rarely

2. I am mindful of my sugar intake and choose healthier alternatives.

- o Often
- o Sometimes
- o Rarely

3. I stay hydrated by drinking plenty of water throughout the day.

- ○ Often
- ○ Sometimes
- ○ Rarely

4. I keep track of the impact of specific food groups on my mood.

- ○ Often
- ○ Sometimes
- ○ Rarely

Mindfulness and Coping Strategies:

1. I practice mindfulness techniques like meditation or deep breathing.

- ○ Often
- ○ Sometimes
- ○ Rarely

2. I have developed healthy coping mechanisms for stressful situations.

- ○ Often
- ○ Sometimes
- ○ Rarely

3. I connect with supportive friends, family, or a therapist when needed.

- ○ Often
- ○ Sometimes
- ○ Rarely

4. I try new coping strategies for managing mood swings.

- ○ Often
- ○ Sometimes
- ○ Rarely

Your Results:

Based on your responses, you may want to focus on the following areas:

- **Identifying triggers:** If you answered "rarely" for questions about trigger awareness, explore common triggers like stress, lack of sleep, and certain foods. Keeping a mood journal can help you identify patterns. Make a mood evaluation section in your diet journal and see if food triggers mood changes like anxiety, depression, and hyperactive mind.
- **Dietary adjustments:** If you answered "rarely" for questions about dietary habits, incorporate omega-3s and magnesium in your diet and limit sugar intake. Consider consulting a nutritionist for personalized advice. Try a different diet approach for two or three weeks and see if there is any impact. Maybe try Keto or Intermittent fasting if that intrigues you and don't forget to keep your diet journal.

- **Mindfulness and coping mechanisms:** If you answered "rarely" for questions about mindfulness and coping strategies, explore techniques like meditation, deep breathing, and journaling. Talk therapy can also be beneficial. Join a chat room or group of like-minded women who will be there to support you through transitions.

Remember, this is just a starting point. Celebrate your strengths and identify areas for growth as you conduct your own personal mood swing symphony.

Disclaimer: This quiz is intended for informational purposes only and does not constitute medical advice. Please consult with your healthcare provider for personalized recommendations.

NOTES:

_____

_____

_____

_____

_____

_____

_____

_____

_____

_____

Chapter 3

Living Well—Diet and Nutrition in Menopause

I want you to imagine strolling into your local supermarket armed with not just a shopping list but a secret treasure map. A map that leads you straight to the aisles filled with foods that could transform your menopausal journey from an unpredictable trek in the dark to a peaceful cruise. Intrigued? You should be.

In this chapter, we're delving deep into the realm of diet and nutrition during menopause. Why? Because what you eat has the power to influence how you feel, from your mood to your energy levels and even those annoying hot flashes. It's time to unlock the mysteries of phytoestrogens, embrace the cooling properties of certain foods, and arm yourselves with the knowledge to make informed choices that support your well-being.

The following pages are all about balance and empowerment. So get ready to embark on a culinary adventure like no other—a journey where the right groceries aren't just items in your shopping cart but powerful tools for living your best life during menopause.

Nutritional Needs during Menopause

It is important to know that there's no one-size-fits-all approach to nutrition during menopause. Listen to your body, embrace the foods that make you feel like a million bucks. Educating yourself on what is good for your body during this transition is essential.

Essential Vitamins and Minerals

First, let's talk about those essential vitamins and minerals that are your new best friends. Picture them as your partners, here to support you through breakouts, hot flashes, mood swings, and everything in between. Here are some great examples (Evans, 2021):

- **Calcium**: Alright, ladies, let's get real. As we age, our bones need a little extra love, especially during menopause when the risk of osteoporosis creeps up like that pesky neighbor's cat. Load up on calcium-rich foods like dairy (if you're into that), leafy greens, and fortified foods. Aim for around 1200 milligrams a day. Your bones will thank you later.
- **Vitamin D**: You know that warm, fuzzy feeling you get from basking in the sunlight? Your body requires vitamin D in order to absorb the calcium you're consuming. But hey, if the sun's playing hide-and-seek, fear not. Fatty fish, fortified foods, and supplements are here to save the day. The recommended dosage for all adults up to age 70 is 600 IU per day.
- **Magnesium**: Say hello to your stress-busting, sleep-promoting pal, magnesium. Menopause can sometimes feel like a never-ending anxiety parade, but magnesium swoops in to keep those cortisol levels in check. Discover

it in seeds, nuts, whole grains, and leafy greens. Magnesium L-Threonate is the most absorbable formula. For women over the age of 31, you should aim for 320 milligrams per day.

- **Vitamin B**: B for "Blast those mood swings away" All the B vitamins are essential but Vitamin B6, in particular, is a superhero for your emotional well-being. Load up on bananas, poultry, fish, and fortified cereals to keep those serotonin levels soaring. For menopausal women, the recommended daily dosage is 1.5 milligrams.
- **Omega-3 fatty acids**: Let's give a round of applause to omega-3s for their inflammation-fighting prowess. These babies are like the firefighters of your body, putting out the flames of hot flashes and joint pain. Flaxseeds, fatty fish, chia seeds, and walnuts are your go-to sources. Aim for 500 milligrams per day.
- **Iron**: Don't let fatigue sneak up on you. Iron is here to keep your energy levels in check and prevent that dreaded menopausal fatigue from crashing your party. Lean meats, beans, lentils, and fortified cereals are your iron-packed pals. If you're Vegan, Vegetarian or just prone to anemia, have your doctor check your iron levels regularly. For women over 50, you should be getting eight milligrams per day.

Balancing Macronutrients

Are you feeling like your pants are suddenly conspiring against you?

So, menopause rolls in like a tornado of hormonal chaos, right? And one of its favorite party tricks is weight gain. But don't worry because we're about to become masters of our macros.

Macros are like the powerhouse of nutrition, here to save the day and keep those maddening pounds at bay. We've got carbs, proteins, and fats ready to fuel our bodies and keep us feeling fabulous.

Now, menopause might throw our metabolism out of whack, but we're not going down without a fight. By balancing our macros, we can manage our weight and keep energy levels soaring.

Here are some fantastic tips to help you conquer menopause weight gain like the empowered woman you are (*Macros for Menopause*, 2023):

- **Be consistent, not perfect:** Menopause is a journey, not a destination, and progress is our ultimate goal. Rather than striving for perfection, let's focus on consistency. Utilize tools like calorie-tracking apps to understand your daily needs and find what works for you. Once you've found your groove, stick to it with unwavering dedication.
- **Boost metabolism:** Revving up your metabolism is key to conquering menopausal weight gain. Incorporate strength training into your routine using resistance bands, Pilates, or free weights. These activities not only build muscle but also stoke your metabolic furnace. And don't forget to prioritize protein-rich foods in your diet —they're the building blocks your body needs to thrive.
- **Rest and manage stress:** The importance of quality sleep and stress management cannot be overstated. Make it a priority to get sufficient, restorative REM sleep each night to support your body's natural processes. Incorporate relaxation techniques such as

deep breathing, meditation, or gentle yoga to keep stress levels in check. Remember, finding your Zen is not just a luxury—it's a necessity for overall well-being.

- **Eat whole, nutrient-dense foods:** Say farewell to processed junk and embrace the nourishing power of whole foods. Load up your plate with colorful fruits, vibrant veggies, and wholesome grains to fuel your body with essential vitamins, minerals, and fiber. By prioritizing nutrient-dense foods, you'll not only support your weight management goals but also enhance your overall health and vitality.

- **Meal prep:** Meal planning is a game-changer on the path to menopause mastery. Take the guesswork out of healthy eating by prepping meals and snacks in advance. Not only does this save time and money, but it also ensures that you always have nutritious options on hand, preventing those impulsive snack attacks that can derail your progress. With meal prep as your ally, staying on track has never been easier.

- **Set goals and track progress:** Rome wasn't built in a day, and neither is menopausal wellness achieved overnight. Be patient with yourself and set realistic, achievable goals along the way. Whether it's increasing your daily step count, mastering a new yoga pose, or simply making healthier food choices, every small victory is worth celebrating. Keep track of your progress, and don't forget to acknowledge how far you've come on your journey to optimal health and vitality.

By embracing these principles—consistency over perfection, prioritizing metabolism-boosting activities, nurturing your body and mind, fueling yourself with nutrient-dense foods, mastering meal prep, and setting and tracking achievable goals—you'll not only navigate menopause with grace and resilience but emerge stronger, healthier, and more empowered than ever before.

Hydration and Menopausal Health

Now, you might be rolling your eyes, thinking, "Really? Again? Water is your big secret?" Well, I'm going to repeat this until the point sinks in. Hydration is not just about drinking some H_2O; it's about giving your body the fuel it needs to navigate the hormonal journey with grace and gusto.

First, discuss the facts. During menopause, hormonal changes can lead to increased sweating and hot flashes. Yep, you're basically your own personal sauna, and that means you're losing precious fluids faster than you can say, "Is it hot in here, or is it just me?"

Staying hydrated is like having a built-in air conditioner for your body. It helps regulate your temperature, keeps your skin glowing (we're talking about that coveted menopausal glow, not just sweat-induced shine), and even boosts your mood (Haskey, 2023). Say goodbye to crankiness and hello to hydration-induced happiness.

The question is, how can we stay hydrated? Step one: drink up, buttercup. Commit to at least eight glasses (64 ounces) of water a day. I know, I know, it sounds like a lot, but trust me, your body will thank you (Haskey, 2023).

But water isn't your only hydration hero. Load up on hydrating foods like fruits and veggies—they're like little water balloons bursting with moisture. Think juicy watermelon, crisp cucumber, and succulent strawberries.

Let's discuss everyone's favorite guilty pleasure: caffeine. I'm not saying you have to give up your morning java, but just be mindful that caffeine can be dehydrating. So maybe swap that third cup of coffee for a refreshing herbal tea or a tall glass of water with a splash of lemon. Your bladder will thank you, too (Haskey, 2023).

And finally, listen to your body. You could be thinking you're hungry when you're actually thirsty. Thirst is your body's way of saying, "Hey, I need some liquid love over here!" So don't ignore it. Keep a water bottle handy wherever you go, and sip, sip, sip away.

Anti-Inflammatory Foods

As estrogen takes a nosedive during menopause, inflammation can increase. And trust me, this is no fun gathering. If left unchecked, this inflammation can wreak havoc on your arteries, organs, and joints, setting the stage for some unwelcome guests like heart disease, arthritis, and even the dreaded dementia (Yeager, 2023c).

Let's ask ourselves how we can help shut down this inflammation.

First, some foods are great at calming inflammation in our bodies. Keep reaching for colorful fresh fruits, crisp veggies, and all those goodies packed with unsaturated fats like avocados, fatty fish, nuts, and olive oil (Yeager, 2023c).

Now, on to diets. Ever heard of the Mediterranean diet? It's like a vacation for your taste buds and your body. The Mediterranean diet is like an anti-inflammatory culinary trip to southern Europe, with a focus on fresh plant foods like veggies, fruits, nuts, and whole grains. It's all about embracing seafood, enjoying just a bit of dairy, poultry, and eggs, and saving red meat for special occasions. Created in the 1960s, it's a delicious way to eat healthy and feel great (Mayo Clinic Staff, 2019b).

Extra virgin olive oil, EVOO as Rachel Ray says, is one of those foods with phenolic compounds that raise the bar with anti-inflammatory action. It is a monounsaturated fat with oleic acid, phytosterols, carotenoids, tocopherols as well as polyphenols. It should star in your daily diet at least once every day without fail.

Olive oil's benefits are not only good for the heart but it also fights diabetes, reduces high blood pressure, helps keep cholesterol under control, strengthens bones, improves gut health and increases those lovely serotonin levels in the brain.

It is important you are mindful of foods that fuel the inflammation fire. We're talking about those ultra-processed refined carbs (looking at you, white bread), sugary beverages (bye-bye, soda), processed meats loaded with preservatives and chemicals (so long, mystery meat), and those sneaky, fat-laden, inflammatory foods fried in oil (we'll miss you, French fries).

Managing Weight with Diet

Shedding those stubborn pounds during and after menopause might feel like trying to win a marathon in flip-flops. Hormone upheaval, stress, and the aging game can team up against you. All is not hopeless. There are some tricks you can employ to outsmart those exasperating pounds during this wild ride.

Healthy Eating Plans

Now, you've probably heard that to shed those extra pounds, you need to create a calorie deficit. Translation? You must consume fewer calories than you burn. Logical, right? Well, sort of.

Here's the scoop: research tells us that during and after menopause, our resting energy expenditure (the calories we burn at rest) takes a nosedive (Spritzler, 2021). Yep, it's like our bodies are saying, "Hey, let's slow things down a bit." Sneaky, right?

Now, I know it might be tempting to go full throttle on a super-low-calorie diet to drop those pounds faster, but hold your horses. Eating too few calories can actually backfire, making weight loss even harder. Plus, it can send your muscle mass packing and put the brakes on your metabolic rate (Spritzler, 2021). Not a good idea.

Sure, those crash diets might give you quick results, but let's be real: Keeping that weight off is like trying to style your hair on a windy day—nearly impossible.

Skimping on calories can also mess with your bones, upping your risk of osteoporosis (Spritzler, 2021). Nobody wants that, right?

So, what's a menopausal maven to do? Fear not, my friends, because I've got some healthy eating plans that'll have you feeling like Wonder Woman in no time.

First, we've got a low-carb diet. Studies have shown that this one's a winner for weight loss, especially when it comes to saying sayonara to that stubborn belly fat. And the best part? You don't have to go full-on keto to see results. A moderate approach can still do the trick (Spritzler, 2021). So cut the carbs that add the weight and cause inflammation like white sugar, white flour, white potatoes, white rice. Count carbs and you'll have fewer pounds to count.

Then, there's the Mediterranean diet. It's not just about sipping wine and soaking up the sun (although that does sound great, doesn't it?). As we discussed, this diet is all about nourishing your body with wholesome goodness while shedding those extra pounds. Plus, it's got the stamp of approval for heart health. Find your favorites and build a routine around these heart healthy, anti-inflammatory foods.

And for our vegan and vegetarian pals. It turns out that ditching meat can do wonders for your waistline and your overall health. Whether you go full-on vegan or opt for a more flexible vegetarian or pescatarian approach, you'll be doing your body a world of good (Spritzler, 2021). Just be aware that you are getting all the necessary vitamins.

Mindful Eating Practices

Let's talk about mindful eating. This is all about balance and nourishment, not deprivation. Mindful eating is all about tuning in to your body's cues, honoring your hunger and fullness, and savoring every delicious bite without judgment.

Can we talk about cravings, those sneaky little diet traps that creep up on us when we least expect it? Whether it's chips, chocolate, or a big bowl of ice cream, we've all been there. And you know what? It's totally okay. Instead of beating yourself up about it, let's get curious. What are those cravings trying to tell us? Maybe our bodies are crying out for some magnesium, or maybe we just need a little pick-me-up to boost our mood. Drink a great big glass of water, then whatever it is, approach it with kindness and understanding. Don't deny yourself that piece of dark chocolate, maybe add a crisp cool apple or a handful of carrot sticks.

Now, onto the good stuff—nourishment. Your ticket to feeling amazing during menopause is great nutrition. Nutrient-packed foods not only fuel our bodies but also help stabilize those pesky hormone fluctuations and keep our energy levels steady throughout the day (Chan, 2020).

And let's not forget about stress. Whether it's through meditation, deep breathing exercises, or simply taking a moment to put your feet up and savor a cup of herbal tea, finding moments of peace and stillness can work wonders for our overall well-being.

Snacking and Metabolism

Oh, the joy of snacking. It's like a mini adventure for your taste buds, right? But here's the thing: snacking during menopause can be a bit of a tightrope walk. Hormonal fluctuations can sometimes lead to those sudden cravings for all things salty, sweet, or just plain comforting. It's like your body's way of saying, "Hey, I need a little pick-me-up"

But before you reach for that family-sized bag of chips or dive headfirst into a pint of ice cream, let's chat about some smarter snacking strategies. Use snacking as an opportunity to nourish your body and keep that metabolism chugging along like a well-oiled machine. We have to be mindful that our metabolism has also slowed during this time, so choosing snacks wisely can help. Reach for the following (Walsh, 2022):

- **Cottage cheese and pitted tart cherries:**
  Consuming protein can help your muscles repair and grow, while protein can improve muscle quality, metabolism, and overall health. Top with tart cherries for their sweet flavor and sleep-promoting powers, thanks to melatonin, a well-known sleep-inducing hormone found in many fruits and vegetables, including tart cherries.

- **Peanut butter and banana:** Bananas are packed with fast-digesting carbs, which can help you relax and boost your metabolism. They're also rich in magnesium, known for calming stress hormones and promoting sleep. The carbs in bananas trigger a chain of internal events that may aid in relaxation. Additionally, the healthy fats in peanut butter can satisfy your brain and body. Just go to this snack sparingly and make it an occasional special treat if it's one of your favorites.
- **Pomegranate juice and 1/2 cup almonds:** Since cinnamon revs up your metabolism (your body burns more energy processing the spice than it does for other foods), why not whip up a warm and comforting mulled cider by simmering pomegranate juice with cinnamon, cloves, and citrus slices? Enjoy it with a handful of almonds for a delightful mix of sweet and salty. These nuts offer tryptophan, magnesium, and an extra boost of protein for your daily intake.

Supplements for Menopausal Support

Yep, we're diving further into the realm of supplements—those little helpers that promise to make this transition smoother than a perfectly mixed margarita on a hot summer day.

Let's start with the basics: Minerals and herbal supplements. These are the essential ingredients in your favorite recipe.

Minerals and Herbal Supplements

- **Flaxseed:** Flaxseed and flaxseed oil could be a savior for women dealing with mild menopause symptoms. Packed with lignans, they have the power to balance those tricky female hormones. However, not all studies agree on their ability to ease pesky vasomotor symptoms such as night sweats (Johnson, 2022).

- **Red Clover:** Many women use red clover for its natural plant estrogens to alleviate their menopause symptoms. Nevertheless, research findings have been inconclusive thus far (Johnson, 2022).
- **Wild Yam:** Certain wild yam species are currently popular as alternatives to hormone therapy for menopause, with pills and creams being made from them. The natural compounds in these yams mimic estrogen and progesterone (Johnson, 2022).
- **Ginseng:** Some research indicates that different types of ginseng may improve the quality of life in menopausal women. Ginseng is associated with mood improvement and better sleep (Johnson, 2022).
- **St. John's Wort**: This treatment is well-known for addressing mild depression, but it may offer an additional benefit for women experiencing menopause. It can improve moods and alleviate troublesome menopausal mood swings (Johnson, 2022).
- **DHEA:** After turning 30, our natural DHEA hormone levels decline. Some research indicates that DHEA supplements may alleviate menopause symptoms such as low libido and hot flashes (Johnson, 2022).
- **Dong Quai:** Dong Quai has long been a popular remedy in traditional Chinese medicine for women's health. A study on its effects on menopausal hot flashes found it to be effective (Johnson, 2022).

Omega 3 Fatty Acids

Let's squash the myth that fat is the enemy. I mean, seriously, who came up with that idea? Fat isn't the villain in this story as long as it's the right kind of fat. And omega-3? Well, it's the champion of the fatty acid world.

Research from way back in 2009 showed that omega-3 could swoop in and reduce the frequency of those bothersome hot flashes (AMC Team, n.d.). So, if you've been avoiding fat, it's time to rethink your strategy.

And get this—omega-3 doesn't stop at hot flashes. Nope, it's like a magical elixir for your whole body, tackling everything from heart disease to diabetes like a boss. Plus, it's got these anti-inflammatory powers that can soothe those frustrating menopause symptoms (AMC Team, n.d.).

Now, when it comes to getting your omega-3 fix, you have options. Sure, you could load up on oily fish, or you could sprinkle some freshly ground flaxseed into your morning smoothie and call it a day. Heck, you could even slurp down some oysters if you're feeling fancy—just make sure you're getting at least two grams a day for best results (AMC Team, n.d.).

But hey, if fish isn't your favorite, no worries! There are plenty of supplements out there just waiting to save the day. Just pop one of those pearls, and you'll be getting all the omega-3 goodness without the fishy aftertaste.

The Role of Phytoestrogens

Let's dive into a topic that might just be your new best friend during menopause: phytoestrogens. Yes, it's a mouthful, but trust me, these little wonders can make a big difference in how you navigate this phase of life.

So, what are phytoestrogens? Think of them as plant-based compounds that can mimic the effects of estrogen in your body. And guess what? They're found in some of your favorite foods. We're talking soybeans, lentils, chickpeas, flaxseeds, and more. Basically, Mother Nature's way of giving you a helping hand during menopause (Karalis et al., 2023).

Now, let's talk about benefits. Phytoestrogens can be your hormone-balancing sidekick. When your estrogen levels start doing a dance, these plant-based buddies step in to help smooth things out. They can alleviate some of those trying symptoms like night sweats, hot flashes, and mood swings. Plus, they might even give your skin that extra glow—who doesn't want that (Karalis et al., 2023)?

But wait, there's more. Phytoestrogens are not just about managing symptoms; they're also your secret weapon for bone health. As we age, our bones can become more fragile, but fear not—phytoestrogens have your back. They can assist in maintaining bone density and lowering the risk of osteoporosis. (Karalis et al., 2023).

In this chapter, we've uncovered the vital connection between diet and overall health, especially during menopause. Eating right is crucial during this phase, but pairing it with the right physical activities can really boost well-being and help manage symptoms. Next up, we'll explore different types of exercises that are especially great for women going through menopause, from strength training to stress-busting activities like yoga and Tai Chi.

Chapter 3 Menopause Management Quiz: Unlocking Your Inner Chef

Ready to embark on a self-discovery adventure and conquer menopause like a champion? Grab your metaphorical magnifying glass and prepare to assess your current strategies. Remember, there's no one-size-fits-all approach, so be honest with yourself and embrace the journey.

Diet:

1. I prioritize whole, unprocessed foods most of the time.

   ○ Often
   ○ Sometimes
   ○ Rarely

2. I incorporate colorful fruits and vegetables into my daily diet.

   ○ Often
   ○ Sometimes
   ○ Rarely

3. I regularly include healthy fats like avocados, nuts, and olive oil in my meals.

   ○ Often
   ○ Sometimes
   ○ Rarely

4. I limit processed foods, sugary drinks, and unhealthy fats.

- ○ Often
- ○ Sometimes
- ○ Rarely

5. I incorporate the Mediterranean diet and its potential benefits.

- ○ Often
- ○ Sometimes
- ○ Rarely

Hydration:

1. I aim to drink at least 8 (8 oz) glasses of water per day.

- ○ Often
- ○ Sometimes
- ○ Rarely

2. I prioritize hydrating foods like fruits and vegetables.

- ○ Often
- ○ Sometimes
- ○ Rarely

3. I limit caffeine intake and choose water or herbal teas when possible.

- ○ Often
- ○ Sometimes
- ○ Rarely

4. I listen to my body's thirst cues and stay hydrated throughout the day.

- o Often
- o Sometimes
- o Rarely

Exercise:

1. I engage in regular physical activity, aiming for at least 30 minutes most days.

- o Often
- o Sometimes
- o Rarely

2. I incorporate strength training exercises to build muscle mass.

- o Often
- o Sometimes
- o Rarely

3. I find activities I enjoy, like walking, swimming, or dancing, to stay active.

- o Often
- o Sometimes
- o Rarely

4. I prioritize getting enough sleep to support my overall health and energy levels.

- ○ Often
- ○ Sometimes
- ○ Rarely

Stress Management:

1. I practice relaxation techniques like deep breathing or meditation to manage stress.

- ○ Often
- ○ Sometimes
- ○ Rarely

2. I prioritize activities that bring me joy and reduce stress, like hobbies or spending time with loved ones.

- ○ Often
- ○ Sometimes
- ○ Rarely

3. I get enough sleep and avoid blue light screens before bed to promote relaxation.

- ○ Often
- ○ Sometimes
- ○ Rarely

4. I seek support from friends, family, or a therapist when needed to manage stress.

- ○ Often
- ○ Sometimes
- ○ Rarely

Understanding Hormones:

1. I have a basic understanding of how hormones fluctuate during menopause.

- ○ Often
- ○ Sometimes
- ○ Rarely

2. I'm aware of common symptoms associated with menopause, like hot flashes, insomnia, weight gain and mood swings.

- ○ Often
- ○ Sometimes
- ○ Rarely

3. I'm comfortable talking to my doctor about my concerns and exploring potential treatment options.

- ○ Often
- ○ Sometimes
- ○ Rarely

4. I'm open to seeking additional information and resources to learn more about menopause.

- ○ Often
- ○ Sometimes
- ○ Rarely

Managing Weight with Diet:

1. I'm aware of the potential impact of menopause on weight management.

- ○ Often
- ○ Sometimes
- ○ Rarely

2. I'm familiar with diet options to lose weight or maintain a healthy weight.

- ○ Often
- ○ Sometimes
- ○ Rarely

3. I'm open to exploring different dietary approaches to support weight management during menopause.

- ○ Often
- ○ Sometimes
- ○ Rarely

Results:

Based on your responses, you might want to focus on:

- **Diet**: If you scored low in the diet section, head to Chapters 2 & 3 for tips on choosing anti-inflammatory foods and exploring the Mediterranean diet.

  - Managing Weight: If you also answered "Rarely" to question 1 in the Managing Weight with Diet section, Chapters 2, 3, and 5 offer specific strategies for healthy weight management during menopause. Consider exploring low-carb, Mediterranean, or vegetarian approaches and incorporating mindful eating practices.

- **Hydration**: Feeling parched? Chapter 4 dives deeper into the importance of staying hydrated and keeping your water bottle handy.
- **Exercise**: Chapter 5 is your guide to finding activities you enjoy and incorporating movement into your daily routine. Don't forget the power of sleep!
- **Stress Management:** Feeling overwhelmed? Chapter 6 provides relaxation techniques and stress-busting strategies to help you find your Zen.
- **Understanding Hormones:** If you're feeling lost, Chapter 7 offers a clear explanation of hormonal changes and empowers you to seek professional guidance if needed.

Remember, this is just a starting point. Celebrate your strengths and explore the chapters that resonate most with you. You've got this, fellow menopause warrior queen.

Disclaimer: This quiz is intended for informational purposes only and does not constitute medical advice. Please consult with your healthcare provider for personalized recommendations.

NOTES:

_____

_____

_____

_____

_____

_____

_____

_____

_____

_____

_____

_____

_____

_____

_____

_____

_____

_____

_____

Chapter 4

Leaping Forward–Physical Activity and Exercise for Menopause

Think of exercise as your personal superpower in the menopause journey. While hot flashes, mood swings, and other symptoms might make you feel like slowing down, this chapter will show you how moving your body can actually turn the tide. From lifting weights to calm, meditative yoga, we'll explore exercises that are not just doable but enjoyable and incredibly effective for your menopausal body. Get ready to leap forward into a world where exercise is your ally in conquering menopause.

Exercise for Hormonal Balance

During menopause, we understand that our body undergoes significant hormonal changes. Estrogen levels decrease, progesterone fluctuates, and various unexpected physical and emotional symptoms make an appearance. Do these experiences resonate with you?

Now, here's where exercise swoops in. When you get moving, your body starts churning out all sorts of feel-good chemicals, like endorphins. Think of them as little happiness friends coursing through your veins, ready to kick some menopausal butt. But it's not just about the mood boost. Exercise also helps balance insulin levels, keeping those blood sugar spikes in check. And don't even get me started on cortisol, a.k.a. the stress hormone. We know too much of this guy can wreak havoc on your system, but regular exercise helps keep him in line (Yüksel et al., 2019).

Let's chat about oxytocin again. That love potion your body brews up when you're cuddling with a puppy or hugging your bestie. Did you know that exercise is like a mini oxytocin factory, pumping out those warm and fuzzy vibes with every squat and lunge? So not only are you getting stronger physically, but you're also giving your mental health a serious boost.

Now, I know what you might be thinking. "But I'm in the throes of menopause, and the last thing I feel like doing is hitting the gym." Trust me, sister, I get it. Some days, just getting out of bed feels like an Olympic feat. But here's the beauty of exercise: it doesn't have to be fancy or complicated; whether it's a brisk walk around the block, a dance party in your living room, or a gentle yoga session, every little bit counts.

Tailoring Exercise for Menopause Symptoms

Ah, the glorious journey through menopause—where the battle against tampons is won, but the war with vaginal dryness rages on. Amid the chaos of hormonal havoc, there shines a beacon of hope: tailored exercise.

It's time to shake off the cobwebs of sedentary living and embrace the exhilarating world of workouts. Bid adieu to the remote control (temporarily, at least) and say hello to a revitalized you.

Why, you ask, is exercise so important during this time? Well, I'm about to drop some knowledge nuggets on you. When those ovaries decide to retire from estrogen production, it's not just about the chin hairs and the memory lapses. No, it's also about dodging the bullets of heart disease, stroke, and osteoporosis. Not exactly the retirement plan we had in mind, right (Cohen, 2022)?

By getting your sweat on, you're not only keeping your ticker ticking and your bones strong, but you're also giving those wicked menopause symptoms a run for their money.

And let's talk about that midlife weight gain. It's about combating the stubborn belly fat that's getting comfortable around your internal organs like an unwelcome visitor. Exercise isn't just about looking good; it's about feeling good and keeping your body in tip-top shape for the long haul.

So, what's the game plan, you ask? Well, it's time to mix it up with a variety of exercises that'll have you feeling fabulous in no time.

Cardiovascular Exercise

Let's talk about heart health, shall we? Did you know that cardiovascular disease is the leading cause of death in women (Lin & Lee, 2018)? Yep, it's a big deal. Engaging in cardio workouts can significantly lower your risk.

Menopause often comes with a side of unwanted weight gain, courtesy of our hormonal rollercoaster. Enter cardio, the ultimate fat-burning machine. Regular cardio sessions rev up your metabolism, torching those pesky extra pounds like a champ (Lin & Lee, 2018).

Now, onto mood and energy levels—two things that can sometimes feel like they're playing hide-and-seek during menopause. Picture this: you finish a refreshing jog or a spirited dance session, and suddenly, you're riding a wave of endorphins, feeling on top of the world. Cardio workouts are a natural mood booster, giving you that extra pep in your step and kicking those mood swings to the curb.

But hey, I get it. The world of cardio can be overwhelming with all its options. So, which one should you go for? Here are a few suggestions:

- **Brisk walking:** Lace up those sneakers and hit the pavement. It's simple and low-impact, just put on those walking shoes and go—no gym membership required.
- **Swimming:** Dive into some laps at your local pool. It's easy on the joints, works every muscle in your body, and leaves you feeling refreshed and invigorated.
- **Cycling:** Whether it's on a stationary bike or cruising through your neighborhood, cycling is a fantastic way to get your legs moving and your heart pumping.
- **Dancing:** Let loose and groove to your favorite tunes. Whether it's salsa, hip-hop, or Zumba, dancing is not only fun but also a killer cardio workout.
- **Interval training:** Short bursts of intense exercise followed by brief rest periods—think sprinting alternated with walking. It's like turbocharging your cardio routine for maximum results in minimal time. (*Cardio Training*, 2022)

Let's explore walking a little further as it's an easy, low-impact exercise that comes with big health benefits. Walking can be done anywhere for any amount of time. Start with 2,000 steps and work your way up to 10,000 steps a day. Keep track with a pedometer. You'll be surprised how quickly those steps turn into miles.

Regular walking not only builds those leg muscles but leads to heart health and fewer chronic diseases as it releases endorphins to enhance your mood.

Kickoff your day with a morning walk and invite a friend or 3 to make it a more social occasion. Alternatively, you can add a short walk to your lunch time routine to shake off the stiffness of sitting in an office all day. After dinner walks are a great way to wind down your day and even help digestion.

Dealing with a busy schedule? Fit in several short walks instead of a long one, or take the stairs at every opportunity.

Remember, consistency is key. Aim for at least 150 minutes of moderate-intensity cardio per week, and watch as your body thanks you with renewed vitality and strength. So, put on your favorite workout gear, crank up the tunes, and show menopause who's boss—one cardio session at a time (*Cardio Training*, 2022).

Strength Training and Bone Health

Let's talk about bone health. Did you know that women are at a higher risk of developing osteoporosis than men? Strength training helps because when you lift weights or do resistance exercises, you're not just toning those muscles; you're also strengthening your bones. And stronger bones mean a lower risk of osteoporosis (*Osteoporosis—Causes*, 2017).

Strength training isn't just about preventing osteoporosis; it's also about building muscle mass. And why is that important? Well, building muscle mass has some serious health benefits. It boosts metabolism, improves balance and coordination (say goodbye to those clumsy moments), and helps maintain a healthy weight.

Research indicates that women going through perimenopause can lose up to 10% of their muscle mass. Interestingly, late peri-menopausal and post-menopausal women are much more likely to experience involuntary muscle loss compared to their pre-menopausal or early perimenopausal counterparts (Ko & Park, 2021).

Muscle loss is no joke. It's not just about losing speed and power; it can also lead to increased insulin resistance, bone loss, fracture risk, and even pave the way for chronic diseases like diabetes and heart disease (Ko & Park, 2021).

The World Health Organization suggests that grown-ups should pump some iron and work those muscles at least twice a week. The CDC also advises including muscle-strengthening activities like weightlifting or push-ups at least two days each week (*Top 10 Things to Know*, 2021).

Strength Training Routines

During menopause, women can include these specific strength training exercises to maintain muscle mass and decrease abdominal fat. (Junggren, 2023):

- **Forearm plank:** Start by lying on the floor or a mat with your forearms flat on the ground, making sure your elbows are directly under your shoulders. Engage your core and lift your body off the floor, keeping your forearms down and your body in a straight line from head to toe. Keep your abs tight and avoid letting your hips rise or drop. Aim to hold this position for 30 seconds. If it hurts your lower back or gets too tough, you can put your knees down to make it easier.

- **One-arm row:** Holding a free weight in your right hand, stand with your feet shoulder-width apart. Bend your knees a bit and make sure to keep those abs engaged. Rest your left hand on your left thigh (or use a chair for extra support if you like). Start with your arm fully extended down. Keep your back straight as you pull the weight up toward your armpit, then lower it back down. Aim for eight to 12 reps, then switch sides and repeat the motion. And remember, no pain, no gain—but don't overdo it.

- **Tricep kickback:** This exercise involves holding a free weight in your right hand and standing with your left leg slightly ahead of your right, with your left knee slightly bent. You can rest your left hand on your left thigh or lean on a chair for support. Keep your tummy muscles tight and back flat, then lift your right elbow until your upper arm is almost parallel with the floor, keeping your elbow close to your body. Straighten your right arm out behind you, making sure to squeeze your triceps as you do so. Return your right hand to the starting position, and remember to strike a pose like a fitness model while doing it. Work up to 3 sets of eight to 12 reps on each side.

Flexibility and Balance Exercises

Imagine you're in a yoga class, gracefully flowing through poses like a majestic warrior princess. With each stretch and twist, you're not only releasing tension but also improving joint health. During menopause, our estrogen levels drop faster than my phone battery. This decline can lead to joint stiffness and even osteoporosis.

Did you know that doing yoga and Pilates can lubricate those joints, increase flexibility, and strengthen bones? It's like giving your body a much-needed oil change (Yeager, 2023b).

Research has proven that yoga can boost muscle strength, flexibility, and overall mobility in individuals dealing with knee osteoarthritis (Deepeshwar et al., 2018). So, strike a pose and let yoga work its magic on those achy knees.

More specifically, yoga poses, such as Downward Dog, Warrior II, Bridge Pose, and Tree Pose, are effective for strengthening the joints (Yeager, 2023b).

Now, let's talk about balance. No, I'm not talking about juggling work, family, and sanity (although, props to you if you are). I'm talking about physical balance. You know, that thing that decides whether we gracefully glide across the room or end up doing a face-plant? As we age, our balance goes as our joints tighten up. Yoga and Pilates are our personal balance coaches. By incorporating poses and exercises that challenge stability, we're not only preventing falls but also boosting confidence. So next time you strut down the street, you'll do it with the swagger of a runway model.

Flexibility and balance aren't just about physical health. They're also about finding equilibrium in our hectic lives. Menopause can feel like riding an emotional rollercoaster with no seatbelt, but practicing yoga and Pilates can help anchor us in the present moment. Suddenly, those mood swings don't seem so daunting when you're flowing through a sun salutation or channeling your inner ballerina.

So, my fabulous menopausal mavens, let's embrace flexibility and balance like the goddesses we are. Whether you're downward-dogging on a yoga mat or pirouetting through a Pilates class, know that you're not just improving your physical health but also nurturing your mind and spirit..

It is important to understand that regular physical activity is a crucial step toward a healthier menopause journey, but it's just one piece of the larger wellness puzzle. While diet and exercise are foundational, exploring holistic and alternative therapies can provide additional support and relief during menopause. These therapies often address not just physical symptoms but also emotional and mental well-being.

Move on to Chapter 5 and discover various holistic and alternative therapies like herbal remedies, acupuncture, and mind-body techniques, offering a comprehensive approach to menopausal health that complements traditional medical treatments.

Chapter 4 Menopause Management Quiz: Find Your Inner Wellness Warrior

Ready to unleash your inner wellness warrior and navigate menopause with confidence? Answer these questions to assess your current strategies and discover personalized tips for a healthier, happier you!

Diet:

1. How often do you choose whole, unprocessed foods over refined options?

- ○ Often
- ○ Sometimes
- ○ Rarely

2. Do you incorporate fruits and vegetables into most of your meals and snacks?

- ○ Often, always a rainbow on my plate!
- ○ Sometimes, I try, but sometimes convenience wins.
- ○ Rarely, I am not a huge fan, but I'm open to exploring.

3. Are you able to manage sugar cravings, especially during hormonal shifts?

- ○ Often, yes, those cravings are my slave
- ○ Sometimes, a little chocolate goes a long way
- ○ Rarely, I'm a slave to sugar

Exercise:

1. How often do you engage in some form of physical activity, like walking, swimming, or dancing?

- ○ Often, at least 3–4 times a week, keeping it moving
- ○ Sometimes, occasionally, when I get the motivation

- ○ Rarely, not really; exercise feels like a chore

2. Do you enjoy trying a variety of exercises or prefer sticking to familiar routines?

- Often, always up for a new challenge
- Sometimes, comfort zone all the way, please
- Rarely, the thought of exercise makes me break into a cold sweat

3. Do you feel confident and supported when it comes to finding exercises that suit your needs and abilities?

- Often, I'm a fitness pro, I got this!
- Sometimes, a little guidance goes a long way
- Rarely, as I'm intimidated by the gym and unsure where to start

Stress Management:

1. Do you have regular practices for managing stress, such as meditation, yoga, or spending time in nature?

- Often, stress doesn't stand a chance in my Zen zone
- Sometimes, I try to unwind, but life often gets in the way
- Rarely, stress is my constant companion, and I don't know how to handle it

2. Do you find it easy to ask for help and support when you're feeling overwhelmed during menopause?

- Often, absolutely! My network is my rock
- Sometimes, because it can be tough to open up, but I'm working on it

○ Rarely, as I tend to bottle things up, not wanting to burden others

Understanding Menopause:

1. Do you feel informed about the physical and emotional changes that occur during menopause?

○ Often, I'm a menopause encyclopedia
○ Sometimes, I have some knowledge, but there's always more to learn
○ Rarely, honestly, I feel confused and overwhelmed by all the changes

2. Do you feel comfortable discussing your menopause experiences with healthcare professionals and trusted friends?

○ Often, open book, baby
○ Sometimes, it can be awkward, but I'm learning to advocate for myself
○ Rarely, as talking about it feels taboo, and I keep things to myself

Results:

Based on your answers, your menopause management journey might benefit from exploring the following:

Diet: If you answered mostly "Sometimes" or "Rarely" now is the time to dive deeper into creating a menopause-friendly diet with recipes and tips. Remember, small changes can make a big difference and the better you feel the more motivated you'll be.

Exercise: If you answered mostly "Sometimes" or "Rarely" look for beginner-friendly exercise options or routines in YouTube videos for variety and resources to help you find activities you enjoy. Everything from chair yoga to wall or floor Pilates, Tai Chi or high-intensity workouts with or without weights. Even some country line dancin' gets you moving. Don't be afraid to experiment and move your body in ways that feel good.

Stress Management: If you answered mostly "Sometimes" or "Rarely" make the time to delve into various stress management techniques like meditation, mindfulness, and relaxation exercises. Remember, prioritizing your well-being is crucial at all life stages, but especially during the transitions of menopause.

Understanding Menopause: If you answered mostly "Sometimes" or "Rarely" go back and review Chapter 1, which provides a comprehensive overview of menopause, its symptoms, and management strategies. Talking to your healthcare professional and connecting with other women going through menopause can also offer valuable support and information.

Remember, this is just a starting point. Celebrate your strengths and explore the chapters that resonate most with you. You've got this, fellow menopause warrior.

Disclaimer: This quiz is intended for informational purposes only and does not constitute medical advice. Please consult with your healthcare provider for personalized recommendations.

NOTES:

_____

_____

_____

Share the Gift of Authentic Well-being

"One of the greatest things you can do to help others is not just to share and give what you have, but to help them discover what they have within themselves to help themselves."

— *Rita Zahara*

Menopause isn't only hot flashes and gaining a little weight. Research shows that low mood, depression, and anxiety can all pose significant problems for women of menopausal age. What's more, although a vast majority of women experience significant symptoms, a relatively small percentage seek help, and the reasons are twofold: they either feel too embarrassed to discuss menopausal symptoms with their doctors, or they believe that these symptoms are "just something you have to put up with."

I have shared various tips such as minding your carb intake, embracing healthy fats, and prioritizing a stress-free life as well as the remarkable benefits of exercise. Many women report feeling more empowered and confident after "the change", and being in your 50s often coincides with hitting career peaks and knowing yourself better than when you were younger. If this book helps add to your sense of confidence, strength, and well-being, please spread the word.

Scan the QR code to leave a review.

Chapter 5

Nurturing Health–Holistic and Alternative Therapies

> " *Healing is a matter of time, but it is sometimes also a matter of opportunity.*
>
> — *Hippocrates*

Embracing the wisdom of Hippocrates, this chapter delves into the realm of holistic and alternative therapies for menopause. It aims to uncover the potential of natural remedies, ancient practices, and modern wellness techniques in rejuvenating and balancing the body and mind during the menopausal transition.

Herbal and Natural Remedies

So, what exactly are herbal medicines? Active ingredients in these products are derived from plant parts, such as leaves, roots, or flowers (*Herbs for Menopause*, 2024). Because I have mentioned herbal remedies that can relieve menopause symptoms in previous sections, let's discuss new ones here (Hill, 2020):

- **Ginkgo biloba:** This is used to give your brain a boost by improving blood flow and nerve transmission, keeping your cognitive health in top shape.
- **Licorice root tea:** Licorice root is another well-liked natural herbal tea that is believed to have the potential to alleviate hot flashes.
- **Valerian root:** Reduces menopausal hot flashes significantly.
- **Passionflower:** It's the go-to for promoting rest and relaxation, perfect for calming an anxious mind before bedtime to help you drift off to sleep.
- **Maca:** Need a boost of energy to tackle your day? Look no further than maca root. This adaptogenic herb can help combat fatigue and enhance your overall sense of well-being and libido, giving you the stamina you need to conquer whatever life throws your way.
- **Sage:** Not just for Thanksgiving dinner, sage is a superstar when it comes to hot flashes. Studies have shown that sage can significantly reduce the frequency and severity of those fiery moments.
- **Chasteberry:** Soothes menopausal symptoms like hot flashes and anxiety with ease.

Integrating Herbs into Everyday Life

Now, I know what you're thinking. "How on earth am I supposed to incorporate all these herbs into my busy life?"

Start by experimenting with herbal teas. Swap out your morning coffee for a soothing cup of sage or red clover tea. Not only will it help alleviate symptoms, but it'll also give you a moment of Zen in your hectic day.

You can also get creative in the kitchen. Add fresh herbs like sage and thyme to your meals for an extra punch of flavor and menopause-fighting power. Whip up a batch of black cohosh-infused soup or sprinkle some maca powder into your morning smoothie for a tasty treat that'll keep you feeling fabulous.

And don't forget about supplements. If you're not getting enough herbs in your diet, consider adding a high-quality supplement to ensure you're reaping all the benefits.

Best Herbal Teas

Let's talk tea, shall we? Picture this: you, cozying up with a warm cup, embracing the magic of herbal remedies to tackle those menopausal moments. Ah, the power of plants.

In the world of herbal teas, we've got some serious allies to help us navigate this journey with grace.

- **Red clover tea:** Packed with plant-derived compounds called phytoestrogens, it's like a natural estrogen that can help balance hormones during menopause. Sipping on this tea might ease hot flashes, night sweats, high cholesterol, high blood pressure, and even bone density issues. This tea has a light floral and fruity taste.
- **Licorice root tea:** It's said to be a hot flash slayer, reducing their frequency and intensity while also giving the body an estrogen-like boost. Not only that, but licorice root may also help with stress management and weight loss. It's like nature's sweet solution in a cup.
- **Dong Quai tea:** Dong Quai, the estrogen-balancing wonder herb. Research suggests it could help reduce hot flashes and night sweats during menopause. In fact, a blend

of Dong Quai and chamomile might slash hot flashes by a whopping 96%! Plus, it could offer relief for pelvic pain and cramps. Just brace yourself for a strong and bitter tea.

- **Valerian root tea:** Valerian root isn't just for the ancient apothecary—it's a natural superpower for sleep and anxiety. Research suggests it could be a game-changer for sleep and hot flashes and even a bone-strengthening ally for those battling osteoporosis. Plus, it's all wrapped up in a cozy, earthy tea package.
- **Ginkgo biloba tea:** This contains phytoestrogens that can help improve hormonal imbalances. But, unlike some other teas, Ginkgo biloba might be just the thing if you're feeling a bit low on energy or finding it hard to concentrate. It's even been said to ease PMS symptoms and lift the mood in pre-menopausal women. Plus, it has a delightful, sweet, and nutty flavor. (Verona, 2022)

Body Therapies

Let's explore some seriously empowering strategies to make this menopause journey smoother than a silk pillowcase on a summer night.

Let's start with body therapies because who doesn't love a little TLC? First up: massage. Picture this: you, lying on a cozy table, soft music playing, and skilled hands working their magic on those tense muscles. Ahh, heaven! Did you know that massage can actually help alleviate those irritating menopausal symptoms? Yup, studies show it can reduce hot flashes, improve sleep quality, and even boost mood by increasing feel-good hormones like serotonin and dopamine (Israel, n.d.). Plus, it's an excuse to treat yourself guilt-free.

Now, let's talk about acupressure. Think of it as acupuncture's no-poke cousin. By applying pressure to specific points on your body, acupressure can help relieve everything from hot flashes to mood swings. It's like a secret weapon against menopausal mayhem. And the best part? You can do it anywhere, anytime— no appointment necessary. So next time you're feeling a bit off-kilter, just press away those woes and get back to slaying the day (Israel, n.d.).

Did you know that hormonal changes during menopause can actually affect your spine and joints? It's true. That's where chiropractic care swoops in to save the day. By gently adjusting your spine, chiropractors can help ease discomfort, improve flexibility, and restore balance to your body. So say goodbye to achy joints and hello to feeling fabulous at any age (McKenna, 2023).

And then there's reflexology—a.k.a. foot magic. Did you know that your feet are a roadmap to your body's inner workings? I'm telling you it's true. By applying pressure to specific points on your tootsies, reflexology can help reduce stress, improve circulation, and even balance those hormonal fluctuations (Muldoon, n.d.). It feels great and talk about putting your best foot forward during menopause!

Last but not least, let's dive into the wonderful world of aromatherapy and essential oils. Did you know that certain essential oils can work wonders for menopausal symptoms?

- **Peppermint:** Picture this: You're feeling hot and bothered, like you're about to melt into a puddle of sweat. Enter peppermint essential oil, the icy-cool superhero of the plant kingdom. Derived from the peppermint plant, this oil packs a refreshing punch that'll make you feel like you just stepped into a winter wonderland. It's your go-to for cooling down those fiery hot flashes, soothing headaches, and even kicking nausea to the curb. Plus, it's like a shot of espresso for your senses, giving you a natural energy boost and sharpening your focus. So when life heats up, reach for peppermint oil and let the cool vibes roll in.

- **Basil:** Stressed out and feeling frazzled? Meet your new best bud: basil essential oil. It's like a breath of fresh air straight from the garden, with a scent that's as calming as a lazy Sunday morning. Derived from the basil plant, this oil is your ticket to tranquility, helping to ease stress and anxiety with just a whiff. And if fatigue's got you down, basil's got your back—it's like a little pick-me-up in a bottle. So when life's got you feeling like you're running on empty, just take a deep breath of basil and let the good vibes flow.

- **Geranium:** This powerhouse oil is supercharger for your hormones, swooping in to save the day during your menstrual cycle, menopause, or any time those hormones start acting up. Derived from the geranium plant, this oil is all about balance, helping to regulate mood swings and keep those emotions in check. And if you're struggling to catch some Z's, geraniums got your back there, too—its calming aroma is a lullaby for your senses, helping you drift off into dreamland with ease. So when you feel like you're on that hormone rollercoaster, reach for geranium oil and let the calm wash over you.

- **Mandarin:** Feeling stressed to the max and in need of a little Zen? Mandarin essential oil to the rescue. This sweet and citrusy oil is like a hug for your nervous system, melting away anxiety and tension with every sniff. Derived from the mandarin fruit, this oil is your ticket to serenity, helping you find your inner calm even on the craziest of days. And if menopause has you feeling like you're about to spontaneously combust, mandarin's soothing properties will have you feeling as cool as a cucumber in no time. So when life's got you feeling frazzled, just take a deep breath and let the stress melt away.

- **Sandalwood:** Are you in need of some serious chill time? Sandalwood essential oil has got your back. This warm and woodsy oil is like a cozy blanket for your soul, wrapping you up in a sense of calm and tranquility. Derived from the sandalwood tree, this oil is your secret weapon against stress, anxiety, and all those vexatious worries that keep you up at night. Just a whiff of sandalwood, and you'll feel like you're drifting off into a peaceful slumber, ready to wake up refreshed and rejuvenated. So when life's got you feeling overwhelmed, reach for sandalwood oil and let the good vibes flow. *(12 of the Best Essential Oils, 2023)*

Energy Healing Techniques

This pivotal phase of your life can have a big impact on your physical, mental, and emotional health, leading to a decline in your overall well-being and self-esteem. Embracing energy healing techniques can make a world of difference.

The Benefits of Reiki

This ancient Japanese healing technique isn't just about a touch-less massage—it's about tapping into the universal life force energy to promote balance and harmony within our bodies. Reiki is like hitting the reset button for your body, mind, and soul. It's like a cosmic massage for your energy but without the need to get undressed. It gently nudges your body back into balance, helping to soothe those ever-present symptoms and restore some peace and tranquility to your life (*Reiki for Menopause*, 2023).

So, what's in it for you besides feeling like you've been wrapped in a cozy blanket of good vibes? Well, let me break it down:

- **Boosted energy:** Reiki can give you that much-needed pep in your step when the fatigue hits harder than a freight train. It's like plugging yourself into a cosmic energy socket and getting recharged.
- **Stress reduction:** Menopause can be a stress fest, am I right? Reiki helps to melt away that tension, leaving you feeling as Zen as a meditation guru on a mountaintop.
- **Hormonal harmony:** With all the hormonal mayhem going on, Reiki swoops in to restore some semblance of balance. It's like having a personal hormone whisperer.
- **Better sleep:** Say goodbye to those restless nights spent tossing and turning like a rotisserie chicken. Reiki can help you drift off into dreamland faster than you can say "snore."
- **Emotional support:** From mood swings to moments of existential crisis, Reiki provides a safe space for you to unload your emotional baggage and emerge feeling lighter and more centered. (*Reiki for Menopause*, 2023)

But does Reiki actually work? Well, let me tell you—the proof is in the eating of the holistic pudding! Studies have shown that Reiki can significantly reduce symptoms associated with menopause (*Reiki for Menopause*, 2023).

Tai Chi and Qigong

So, Tai Chi—it's a gentle dance party from ancient China. Instead of busting moves to the latest hits, you're gracefully practicing slow, deliberate movements. Picture yourself as a martial arts master, except without the intense combat, because who needs all that stress?

There are different flavors of Tai Chi, like Chen, Yang, and Wu, each with its own unique style. But despite the differences, they're all about one thing: getting your mind and body to shake hands and become besties (Newton & Snyder, 2021).

It's all about that mind-body connection.

And then there's Qigong—think of it as Tai Chi's chill cousin. While Tai Chi is like a carefully choreographed ballet, Qigong is more like a casual stroll in the park. It's all about simplicity.

Qigong (pronounced "chee" "gong") has been around for over 4,000 years—It's the original holistic health practice, using gentle movements, breathing exercises, and even a sprinkle of meditation to keep your qi flowing smoothly (Newton & Snyder, 2021).

Tai Chi and Qigong help with stress relief and overall well-being. They both aid in fighting inflammation and ease aches and pains (Newton & Snyder, 2021).

Meditation and Energy Flow

Yoga and meditation—the dynamic duo that can sprinkle some serious mind-body magic into your life, especially during this chaotic journey of hormones.

So, we all know yoga and meditation are like the super forces of the wellness world. They flex muscles, calm minds, and even help shed a few pounds—what's not to love? But what's their special power when it comes to perimenopause, menopause, and post-menopause?

Imagine that you're striking a yoga pose, gracefully flowing from one position to the next. What you may not realize is that those twists and bends are sending fresh blood deep into your organs—think kidneys, thyroid, and even that quirky pituitary gland hanging out in your brain. And hey, if we're treating our thyroid right, it's like giving a thumbs-up to our body temperature regulation, potentially giving those hot flashes the cold shoulder (*Yoga, Meditation*, 2019).

Yoga isn't only about striking a powerful pose; it's about finding your Zen within the chaos. It's about tuning into your body, quieting the mind, and giving your nervous system a much-needed breather. And let's not forget the mental gymnastics involved—concentrating on breathing into a graceful Downward Dog helps you forget about everything else (*Yoga, Meditation*, 2019).

And meditation? It's a soothing balm for your frazzled nerves. Imagine sinking into a state of tranquility, letting go of the day's worries, and allowing positive vibes to flow through you like a gentle stream. It's like taking a timeout for your brain, calming anxious thoughts, and giving your restless limbs a well-deserved break.

Sure, finding time to meditate every day might seem like a huge task when life is throwing a million things your way. You can sneak in a quick session at the end of your yoga practice or tune into a guided meditation podcast while you're cooking dinner or commuting to work (not while driving). Five minutes here, ten minutes there—before you know it, you'll be a meditation master, and benefits? They'll stack up faster than a pile of old magazines.

Guided Imagery

Picture yourself in a serene setting, like a tranquil beach. Feel the gentle waves, smell the salty air, and imagine the soft sand between your toes. How does the breeze feel against your skin?

This is an example of guided imagery in action, and taking short, regular breaks like this might help you feel more relaxed. Here are a few ways it can alleviate menopause symptoms (Migala, 2023):

- **Mood boost:** Ever notice how a stroll through nature can magically melt your worries away? Guided imagery taps into that same Zen vibe. It's like taking a mini-vacation in your mind so, even if you're stuck in the daily grind, you can still find moments of serenity wherever you are.
- **Stress relief:** Life gets messy, especially during menopause. Guided imagery can be your trusty stress-buster sidekick. Once you've mastered the art of mental escapism, you can whip out your serene sanctuary whenever stress comes knocking. Whether it's first thing in the morning to kickstart your day or last thing at night to wind down, this practice is your ticket to keeping those negative thoughts at bay.

Cultivating a Healthy Microbiome for Menopause

Your gut is the center of a whole universe of bacteria and microbes that can make a huge difference in how you experience menopause.

Understanding the Gut-Health Connection

So, why does your gut matter during menopause? You see, your gut is like a second brain, influencing everything from your mood to your immune system. And guess what? It's also connected to your hormonal balance. Yep, those trying hormones can throw your gut out of whack, leading to all sorts of fun stuff like bloating, irregularity, and even affecting mood swings. Studies show that estrogen, especially, has a big influence on the makeup of the gut microbiome, and a change in estrogen levels can affect it. So, taking care of your gut is crucial for smoother sailing through menopause (Hodgkinson, 2023a).

Probiotic Foods and Supplements: What's the Deal?

What's the difference between prebiotics and probiotics? In a nutshell, you want both because probiotics are the foods you eat (think natural yogurt) and supplements you take that contain live microorganisms necessary to maintain or improve the "good" bacteria, and prebiotics (think garlic and apples) are the foods you eat that feed those good bacteria.

Now, onto the good stuff—specifically about probiotics. These little darlings are the superheroes of your gut, helping to keep everything in balance. You can find them in delicious foods, not only yogurt but also kefir, sauerkraut, and kimchi. Or, if you're not a fan of fermented foods, you can always opt for a high-quality probiotic supplement. Probiotics can help replenish the good bacteria in your gut, keeping your microbiome happy and healthy during menopause (Luque, 2020).

Diet's Impact on Gut Health

Next up, let's talk, again, about what you're putting on your plate. Your diet plays a massive role in the health of your gut, especially during menopause. Digestive issues such as constipation, diarrhea, bloating, or gas could be a sign that your gut microbiome is out of balance. Load up on fiber-rich fruits and veggies, whole grains, and lean proteins. These goodies feed the good bacteria in your gut, helping them flourish and keep those unwanted gastrointestinal symptoms at bay. Oh, and don't forget to hydrate, hydrate, hydrate. Minimum two quarts or liters daily, if you recall. Water is essential for maintaining a happy gut and much more.

Strategies for Gut Wellness

So, what can you do to keep your gut in tip-top shape during menopause? Well, aside from concentrating on probiotic-rich foods and filling your plate with fiber, there are a few other tricks:

- **Cut out unhealthy things:** Some foods can disrupt the balance of good bacteria in your gut, causing inflammation and affecting your gut health. To maintain a healthy gut, remember to avoid foods with refined sugar and flour, processed foods, artificial and plant sweeteners, alcohol, processed meat, excessive red meat, refined oils, and fried foods. Remember, a healthy gut leads to a healthier you (Hodgkinson, 2023a).
- **Plant foods:** Research suggests that opting for a colorful variety of plant foods, like fruits, veggies, nuts, seeds, and whole grains, can lead to a more diverse community of gut microbes. So, the more, the merrier (Hodgkinson, 2023b).

- **Sleep:** You know that a good night's sleep is mandatory for our bodies, repairing and resetting us for the next day's adventures. Skimping on sleep can turn us into stress monsters, wreaking havoc on our hormones and gut health. Embracing a bedtime ritual, steering clear of late meals or midnight snacks, cutting down on screen time, and unwinding with relaxation techniques can all contribute to enhanced quality of sleep. And for those of us navigating menopause, addressing its symptoms every way possible can be the key to reclaiming peaceful nights.

- **Prebiotic foods:** Think of prebiotics as the ultimate gut fertilizer for probiotics, the normal microflora we all need. Prebiotics are the VIP treatment for good gut microbes, providing nourishment and helping them thrive. These special foods, like asparagus, garlic, bananas, apples, legumes, and oats, are high in fiber and indigestible by the body, so they head straight to the colon, where they become a feast for gut microorganisms. As a result, they churn out highly beneficial short-chain fatty acids, which do wonders for our metabolism, inflammation levels, and immune system. However, not everyone can handle this VIP treatment, and for some, it can lead to gut health problems. If you have SIBO (Small Intestinal Bacterial Overgrowth) or FODMAPS intolerance, prebiotics are not recommended. FODMAPS are fermentable oligosaccharides, disaccharides, monosaccharides and polyols, which are short-chain carbohydrates (sugars) that the small intestine absorbs poorly. Wheat, garlic and onions lead the list.

- **Polyphenols:** These plant compounds are the kings of the food world. They have antioxidant powers, promote good gut bacteria, and even take down bad microbes. You can find these mighty polyphenols in delicious foods like berries, nuts, seeds, beans, and olives.

- **Wholegrains:** These foods bulk up your stools, providing fiber and nourishment for the good gut microbes. Think of them as the superchargers of your digestive system. Great wholegrains to include are rice, corn, oats, and bulgur wheat.
- **Reduce stress:** Stress doesn't just mess with our minds; it also impacts our bodies. In fact, one study of over 700 people revealed that 66% of those with gut health issues take a hit when they're feeling anxious (Hodgkinson, 2023b). It's crucial to dig deep and figure out what's causing the stress in order to tackle it. Sharing the mental load, practicing meditation and mindfulness, taking regular breaks, and showing yourself some kindness can all help. And if things get really tough, don't hesitate to seek professional help.
- **Move that body:** Just like sitting around too much can mess with your gut bacteria, pushing yourself too hard can do the same. So, finding the right balance is crucial. Engaging in regular, gentle-to-moderate exercise and muscle-strengthening workouts can do wonders for your gut health and keep things moving smoothly (if you'll forgive the pun).
- **Fermented foods:** These sharp and tasty foods are like a bustling city for good bacteria. They're packed with probiotics that can help populate your gut with healthy microbes and promote a diverse gut microbiome. Some top-notch examples of these probiotic-packed foods are kefir, kimchi, kombucha, and sauerkraut. (Hodgkinson, 2023a)

Get into the habit of routinely doing the things that will help naturally balance your hormones:

1. Get quality protein for the amino acids your body can't make
2. Eat healthy fats
3. Be aware of your gut health
4. Reduce your sugar consumption
5. Exercise regularly
6. Lower stress
7. Get high quality REM sleep

It is vital to take care of our internal health while traveling the menopause journey. These holistic approaches can help you do just that. Next, we will look at the importance of external support systems. A strong community and support network are equally crucial in the menopause journey.

While individual health practices are essential, the role of social and emotional support should not be underestimated. In the next chapter, we will explore the power and importance of building a supportive community during menopause.

Chapter 5 Menopause Management Quiz: Unlocking Your Inner Herbalist

Ready to embrace the wisdom of Hippocrates and explore the world of natural remedies for menopause? Buckle up, goddess! This quiz will help you assess your current arsenal and discover new tools to combat your menopausal foes with humor and holistic power.

Herbal Allies:

1. How often do you brew up a cup of herbal tea, feeling the magic of plants soothe your soul?

- Often, daily ritual—I'm a tea-drinking superstar
- Sometimes, occasionally, when I remember
- Rarely, never really considered it

2. Do you find exploring new herbs and their benefits exciting, or do you stick to your tried-and-true favorites?

- Often, always open to new plant friends
- Sometimes, I'm comfortable with what I know
- Rarely, herbs sound a bit witchy, not for me

3. Do you ever incorporate fresh herbs into your cooking, adding a dash of flavor and menopause-fighting power?

- Often, my kitchen is an herb garden
- Sometimes, for special occasions
- Rarely, convenience wins, I mostly use dried spices

4. Have you considered adding herbal supplements to your routine for a concentrated dose of goodness?

- Often, already got my herbal apothecary stocked
- Sometimes, intrigued, but unsure where to start
- Rarely, supplements feel a bit risky, I prefer natural foods

Body Magic:

1. How often do you treat yourself to a relaxing massage?

- Often, at least monthly pampering session—self-care queen
- Sometimes, occasionally, when I have a special occasion
- Rarely, massage? More like "massage, who has time for that?"

2. Have you ever tried acupressure, applying gentle pressure to unlock your inner balance?

- Often, I'm a self-acupressure pro
- Sometimes, open to trying it, but unsure where to start
- Rarely, sounds a bit too woo-woo for me

3. Have you considered chiropractic care to keep your spine aligned and your body in harmony?

- Often, regular adjustments are my secret weapon
- Sometimes, I've heard good things, but haven't tried it
- Rarely, chiropractic sounds scary, I'll stick to traditional medicine

4. Do you ever indulge in reflexology, letting your feet be your roadmap to relaxation?

- Often, foot pampering is a must
- Sometimes, intrigued, but haven't had the chance
- Rarely, foot massages are fine, but reflexology sounds weird

5. Are you familiar with the power of essential oils, harnessing nature's scents for mood and symptom relief?

- Often, my diffuser is my best friend
- Sometimes, I've heard of them, but haven't explored much
- Rarely, essential oils sound interesting, but I'm worried about safety

Energy Awakenings:

1. Have you ever experienced Reiki, tapping into universal energy to promote balance and peace?

- Often, Reiki regular, feeling the good vibes flow
- Sometimes, curious about it, but haven't taken the plunge
- Rarely, Reiki sounds a bit mystical, not for my practical mind

2. Do you engage in any other energy healing techniques like meditation or yoga to quiet your mind and nurture your soul?

- Often, my inner Zen master is always on the mat
- Sometimes, I'm open to trying new practices
- Rarely, meditation sounds boring, and yoga seems too intimidating

3. Have you ever tried Tai Chi or Qigong, gentle movements that promote stress relief and well-being?

- Often, flowing like a master, channeling my inner warrior

- Sometimes, curious about trying them, but haven't explored
- Rarely, these practices seem a bit too slow-paced for me

Expanding Your Horizons:

Mind-Body Magic:

- Consider exploring yoga and meditation for stress relief, improved sleep, and a deeper connection to your body. Stop eating/drinking at least two hours before bedtime. Turn off all screens. Enjoy some soothing music. If your mind is racing about the many things you have to do tomorrow, make a list then give yourself permission to put it away until tomorrow. Put a little lavender in your essential oil diffuser for a restful sleep. Set the room temperature to a comfortable setting. Wash your face, brush your teeth, and pamper yourself with a hydrating lotion.

Guided Imagery:

- Learn how to use guided imagery for a quick mental escape and mood boost. Chapter 5 provides tips and suggestions for creating your own serene sanctuary. Recognize that sleep hygiene is a real thing. Don't settle for falling asleep on the couch in the middle of a Netflix binge and waking up stiff and unrested.

Gut Wellness:

- Discover the crucial role your gut plays in menopause and how to nourish it with probiotics, prebiotics, and other dietary strategies. Cultivate a happy gut microbiome with both prebiotics and probiotics. Discard all those boxes and bags of highly processed foods in the pantry and say no to inflammatory food like "The Whites." No white sugar, No white flour, No white potatoes, No white rice. Go even further to support your digestive system by eliminating fried foods. If you can't go 100% fried food free, try to limit fried options to only once a week and notice how you feel after eating the fried stuff. In some cases, dairy may be problematic, so try going dairy-free for two or three weeks and note in your food journal how your body reacts when you eat dairy again and what kinds of dairy are the worst culprits.

Building a Support Network:

- Remember, you're not alone. Make it your mission to support other women and build your personal support network. Remember, we're all going through some stages of hormonal fluctuations, whether we recognize it or not. Knowing why you feel the way you feel and that you're not the only one going through these changes, sharing solutions that work for you, and hearing new information are all encouraging ways to improve your life journey.
- As we move into Chapter 6 we'll talk more about building a support network.

Disclaimer: This quiz is intended for informational purposes only and does not constitute medical advice. Please consult with your healthcare provider for personalized recommendations.

NOTES:

Chapter 6

Embracing Community—Building a Support Network for Menopause

> " *The best preparation for tomorrow is doing your best today.*
>
> — *Jackson Brown*

I n this chapter, we delve into the power of connection, empathy, and shared experiences. We'll explore how embracing a supportive community can be the cornerstone of a smoother, more enriching menopause journey.

Recognizing the Importance of Support

Menopause is a major life change that brings a lot of physical, emotional, and social shifts. It's a time when we can really benefit from the connection and support of others who are navigating or have gone through it.

Emotional and Psychological Benefits

We are all well aware of how menopause can feel like it throws our emotions into a blender, leaving us feeling uncertain most days. Having a supportive community gives us a safe space to vent and get some high-fives of validation. Knowing you're not alone in this wild ride is pretty empowering.

Sharing Experiences and Advice

Talking with other menopausal women gives us a space to share common experiences, from the physical symptoms and emotional challenges to the lifestyle adjustments that come with this journey. This shared understanding fosters empathy and reminds women that we don't have to face this transition alone.

Building a Community

Menopause has been wrapped in secrecy for too long, making us feel like we're in the dark about what's coming. By creating a community, we're smashing through the silence and offering a safe, open space to share experiences, worries, and wisdom. It's all about building a place where we feel heard, acknowledged, and supported.

A community is a treasure trove of education and empowerment. It's where we swap knowledge, resources, and tips we've picked up from our own experiences. Whether it's new kinds of self-care strategies or symptom management tricks, this information exchange gives us the power to make smart choices about our health and well-being.

Communities centered on menopause often result in deep and forever friendships. These connections can outlast menopause, offering ongoing support, fun, and shared experiences for years to come. Having a group of friends who truly understand the ups and downs of menopause can be a priceless.

Online and Offline Support Groups

Support groups for menopausal women provide a great chance to team up and tackle challenges together. From finding ways to combat brain fog to sharing tips for better sleep, these groups offer a space for us to support each other and come up with creative solutions. By working together, we can tap into a wealth of knowledge and diverse viewpoints, making the journey through menopause a bit more manageable and even enjoyable.

Support groups can be like a magnet for expert advice and professional support. By bringing in healthcare pros, therapists, nutritionists, and other specialists to answer questions and share their wisdom, the community can level up its resources and offer invaluable information to members.

Within support groups, we can swap resources, share book and podcast recommendations, and discuss all sorts of great online tools. This collaborative knowledge-sharing guarantees we have the resources to help us to come out the other side of this menopausal adventure better than ever.

Nurturing Family and Friendships

Navigating menopause is juggling a circus of physical, emotional, spiritual, and mental changes all at once. Like trying to keep all the plates spinning while riding a unicycle. Expressing what's going on can feel like trying to describe a complicated magic trick… in latin—it's personal and puzzling because it is hard for us to understand most days.

Research shows that having supportive family and friends can make this wild ride feel more like a cozy tea party (Donsky, 2024). Menopause can be challenging, but with the right support, it doesn't have to feel like it's insurmountable or never ending.

Communication Strategies

One crucial aspect is the ability to express emotions openly. It's important to be able to discuss our experiences and feelings without fear of judgment while also having family members who are willing to listen and offer assistance. Tell your family and friends that the right questions to ask are "How can I help you at this moment?" or "Can you tell me how you're feeling right now?" Doing so will show that they care and want to support you. If they haven't been through something similar, themselves, they won't have a clue how to act or how to best help you at any given time.

Can you think of a time in your life when a friend or family member confided in you about an illness or tough time they were going through? For example, maybe your spouse or partner was diagnosed with chronic depression. Did you reach for any information you could get your hands on to better understand it?

Knowledge is power, and sharing the importance of understanding menopause with your loved ones shows that they care. Menopause is complicated, impacting the body, emotions, mind, and social life. By trying to understand it, they can better support you through this journey.

Maggie's Story

A busy mom of three and a career woman, Maggie had convinced herself she just wouldn't give menopause the attention it may have deserved. "Who has time for all this nonsense?" she would say. While her friends would be complaining about the myriad of symptoms, she was pushing through without a word. A few years in, she was hit with incredible cognitive decline. A professional accountant she felt this most at work, making mistakes in a job in which she took incredible pride. Unable to sleep more than three hours at a time, the fatigue was taking a toll. She tried speaking to her male boss, who was well into his 60s. Not surprisingly, she wasn't met with a lot of sympathy. She then tried speaking to her family doctor, another male pushing retirement age. What she discovered was that both men, whom she deemed superior, in fact, treated her as less. She was told she was simply "overdoing it" and needed to take it easy. Despite her pleas that this wasn't depression, she was given an antidepressant by her doctor.

As the weeks went on, her symptoms worsened. Her family always found these "episodes" hilarious, often met with comments like "Hey, Mom, are we going to lose our phone today?" or "Dear, I put your keys right by the door so you won't have to spend hours looking for them... again." If she seemed flustered and unable to find a word, they would burst into laughter. The last straw came during Thanksgiving dinner when she forgot the dinner rolls were in the oven, as they burned to a crisp. Laughter erupted, and she burst into tears. She left the room and locked herself in the bathroom, sobbing. Now, with concerned looks on their faces, they knew they had gone too far. A family meeting was held the next week, and she asked them all to just listen. She explained that she hadn't felt heard in years, not by her boss, her doctor, or even her family. She wanted them to ask themselves how they would feel if one day they felt they couldn't do their job or remember the word for car. She talked about how terrified, frustrated, and angry she was. Wrapping her in love and support, they apologized and said they now understood their new roles in her life. Her husband would accompany her to appointments until she found the right doctor who would take her symptoms seriously. She would meet with Human Resources and discuss what she needed at work. Her family would listen when she communicated her needs. Maggie's story illustrates the importance of talking to those around us, explaining clearly what you need and from whom. This can only help.

Setting Boundaries and Expectations

Boundaries are like the bouncers of our personal club, deciding who and what gets in. We need to take charge and set those boundaries ourselves. It's all about what behaviors we're okay with and what we won't put up with. For instance, if someone starts being dismissive of you or your opinions, you have every right to leave that conversation. If a friend or family member starts disrespecting your, very real, menopause symptoms, you have the power to walk away. That's your boundary, and you have every right to enforce it.

Rather than seeing boundaries as a means of exclusion, they actually serve to roll out the red carpet for the high-quality people who benefit your life.

Throughout our lives, we often make numerous sacrifices to ensure our families are well taken care of, leaving little time to focus on ourselves. Our hormones play a big role in this, driving us to reproduce and care for children and others. It's an evolutionary instinct that can blur or even erase personal boundaries. Yes, our hormones have quite an influence.

So, when menopause comes knocking and the hormones start to create havoc in our bodies, a lot of us find ourselves feeling a bit angry and frustrated. As the hormonal fog clears, it's no surprise we're left wondering, "Hey, what about me?"

Menopause is the perfect time to take a good look at ourselves, our lives, and our families. It's a good opportunity to reset boundaries that will help us lead a more fulfilling life and set the goals that will truly serve us for the next stage of our journey.

This is the right time to define our boundaries around family, work, home, and friends.

The big question is, how do we set boundaries?

- **Where do I need boundaries?:** Take a close look at areas of your life where things feel out of balance, a relationship seems off track, or your ability to communicate with someone has hit a roadblock.
- **What boundaries are mandatory?:** Make a firm decision to set boundaries in those areas of your life. And if it helps, jot them down.
- **Set one boundary at a time:** Keep it simple.
- **Keep emotions out of it:** You should set boundaries when you're feeling calm and content, not when you're angry, lonely, or overtired. Like trying to fly a kite with no wind—it's just not the right time.
- **Re-evaluate:** Be ready to tweak them if they're not working for you or aren't meeting your needs. And remember, flexibility is key.
- **Be realistic:** If you set impossible boundaries, you're basically asking for trouble.
- **Expect setbacks:** Just because you have a chat about boundaries with someone doesn't mean they'll be easily implemented. People might revert to old behaviors and need a gentle reminder. Practice this phrase "That doesn't work for me."

Engaging in Shared Activities

So, how do we keep the flames of friendship burning bright during menopause? Well, let's start with shared activities. Instead of letting those unpleasant symptoms get the best of us, why not turn them into opportunities for fun and bonding? Here are a few ideas:

- **Sweat it out together:** Literally! Gather your gal pals or family for a workout session or a brisk walk in the park. Exercise not only helps alleviate menopausal symptoms but also releases those feel-good endorphins, leaving you with a smile on your face.
- **Cook up a storm:** Embrace the power of good food and good company by hosting a cooking night. Whip up some delicious, hormone-balancing recipes together while swapping stories and laughter. Who knows? You might just discover a new favorite dish.
- **Spa day, anyone?** Treat yourselves to a pampering session at home or splurge on a day at the spa. Massages, facials, and relaxation are just what the doctor ordered to combat stress and promote overall well-being.
- **Get crafty:** Channel your inner creativity by diving into a DIY project or an art class. Whether it's pottery, painting, or knitting, getting crafty together can be both therapeutic and loads of fun.
- **Game night extravaganza:** Dust off those board games or fire up the console for a night of friendly competition. Game nights are a fantastic way to unwind, let loose, and bond over some healthy rivalry.

Understanding and Empathy

We all have days on this journey where we don't feel understood by those who love us most. Needing empathy and understanding from friends and family is crucial.

We need to feel confident enough to express our feelings, even when we lose our keys or can't find our glasses. It's important to help each other out in those moments. We can laugh about it later, but it's important to know when it's okay to joke and when it's not.

It's crucial to remember that we're not looking to be "fixed." That just makes us feel helpless or like a burden. We're simply seeking support, understanding, and empathy from our loved ones. It's totally fine to share a laugh with us, just not at our expense.

It's a big help when our friends and family realize that our explosive emotions aren't aimed at them. We get that it can be pretty frustrating and confusing to deal with.

Communication is key for us. Being able to chat with our partner, kids, or friends about our feelings and feeling heard can be life-changing. Just like everyone else, we want to feel cared for and supported by our loved ones.

Shannon's Story

Shannon's story (not her real name) is not to scare you but to empower you. Why? Because she had no idea this could happen to her. When she was 52, she had a heart attack. Otherwise healthy, she didn't smoke or drink alcohol, and wasn't overweight. Yet, there she was, in the emergency room, suffering a heart attack.

She had never been so terrified. She grabbed the nurse's arm, looked her in the eye, and said emphatically, "Do not let me die!"

The next eight days in the hospital they tried to figure out what the cause was. No blockages, no build-up, and one male doctor after another tried to convince her this was a "fluke" of sorts and she had nothing to worry about.

She knew this couldn't be the case.

She continually told them she had been experiencing menopausal symptoms for the last year, and they were much worse in the last six

months. As part of this, heart palpitations were waking her from her
sleep.
Without fail, they would all look at her while she talked, flip
through her chart, and, without missing a beat, tell her it was likely
anxiety. It was frustrating and exhausting. It took six months to track
down a female cardiologist, and with one look at Shannon's blood-
work, she knew the problem.
Shannon was dangerously anemic, and her estrogen levels were extremely
low. This was a combination that also made her platelets low. A recipe
for a heart attack. Six months after being on iron supplements, blood
thinners, and a cardiac rehab program, she felt like a new woman.
If you find yourself in medical distress and you aren't being listened
to, don't give up. Keep pushing because you deserve to be heard.

Professional Support and Counseling

It's essential to recognize that while menopausal symptoms are as common as birds chirping in the morning, it doesn't mean you have to tough it out alone. Sure, a few mood swings here, a sprinkle of crying outbursts there, but if these symptoms start staging a full-on takeover of your life, it's time to wave the white flag and seek some expert advice.

So, when should you pick up that phone and make that appointment? Well, if your daily routine resembles an unbearable rollercoaster ride through symptom city, and you find yourself unable to function at work or feeling like a regular on the unwell express, it's a clear sign to dial up your doctor. If you're experiencing unexpected anxiety that's turned the dial up to 11—it's another red flag to get some professional insight (Cotsen, 2018).

Therapy can be your backstage pass to navigating the intense emotions we all experience. Chatting with a therapist about how menopause is rocking your world can help you unearth deeper emotions you might not have even realized were there, buried under layers of life's chaos.

Think of menopause as your grand entrance into a new chapter of life. Sure, it's the end of one era—the baby-making factory is closing up shop—but it's also the start of something exciting. No more monthly cycles, birth control debates, or worrying about that infamous biological clock.

But hey, just because the fertility factory is closing doesn't mean the fun has to end. It's time to embrace the joys of motherhood, explore your sexuality with renewed vigor, dive into new relationships, and relish in the freedom to pursue your passions without undesirable periods butting in.

Now, finding the right therapist is key. Just like shopping for the perfect pair of shoes—sometimes, you have to try a few pairs before you find the right fit. Take your time, explore different therapy styles, and don't settle until you find a connection that's comfortable.

Menopause and Life Coaches

Life coaching isn't just about setting goals and achieving dreams (although that's part of it). It's like having a wise, supportive, certified sidekick by your side, equipped with all the tools you need to navigate menopause.

So why should you consider recruiting a life coach for this wild journey? Let me break it down for you:

- **Stress-buster:** Menopause is like a stress bomb going off in your body. A life coach can swoop in with mindfulness tricks and stress-busting techniques to help you ride the waves of change with ease.

- **Goal-getter:** Feeling like you've lost control? Not on the life coach's watch. They'll help you set clear, achievable goals to reignite your sense of purpose and direction.
- **Emotional anchor:** Mood swings turning you into a human tornado? A life coach provides a safe harbor to vent, strategize, and conquer those emotional loop de loops.
- **Body boost:** Say goodbye to the menopause belly blues. Your life coach will team up with you and your new approach to diet and exercise to whip your body into shape with exercise routines and healthy eating habits.
- **Relationship rescue:** Is Menopause putting a strain on your relationships? Your life coach is here to help you navigate the sometimes-stormy seas of communication and connection.
- **Confidence crafter:** Hormones wreaking havoc on your self-esteem? Let your life coach be your cheerleader, boosting your confidence and self-love.
- **Time tamer:** Juggling a million things at once? Your life coach will teach you the art of time management and prioritization so you can slay your to-do list like a boss.
- **Support squad:** Feeling like you're on this journey alone? Your life coach will help you build a tribe of supportive friends and professionals to lean on when the going gets tough. (Crossett, 2023)

Finding the right life coach is key. Look for someone who specializes in menopause or women's health, someone you connect with, and who comes armed with the proper credentials.

Leveraging Technology for Support

Traversing this journey in the modern world does have its perks. Why not lean into some high-tech advances to make things run a bit smoother?

Online Forums and Social Media

Ever found yourself waking up at 3 a.m., drenched in sweat, wondering if you're the only one going through this madness? News flash: you're not. Enter online communities and forums dedicated to menopause.

Here are the top five menopause forums, communities, discussion, and message boards for 2024:

1. **Menopause Matters Forum:** Providing accurate information about menopause and treatment options, an independent site led by clinicians strives to offer valuable insights.
2. **Menopause ChitChat:** Crafted with your needs in focus. Join other women to converse about symptoms, challenges, and remedies.
3. **Reddit » Menopause:** Reddit consists of communities centered around people's interests. This one specifically centers around women and menopause.
4. **Jo's Cervical Cancer Trust Forum » Coping with Menopause:** In the "Coping with menopause" category, dealing with menopause due to cervical cancer treatment or cell changes can be challenging, whether it

has recently begun or you are still experiencing it. This category is designed for you.

5. **Live Better With Community » Menopause:** The question and answer hub provides a platform to access free expert advice from qualified health professionals in the convenience of your own home. (*Top 10 Menopause,* 2024)

Menopause Tracking Apps

Tired of menopause symptoms crashing your party? Fear not, because there's an app for that. Yep, you heard it right. These apps are like your personal menopause cheerleaders, connecting you with doctors, offering community support, and even handing out prescriptions for those unrelenting symptoms. Plus, they've got great trackers to monitor all of your symptoms, making it easier to chat with your healthcare team about what's been going on. Here is the cream of the crop (fees current as of publishing):

- **Evernow:** It's got the celebrity stamp of approval and a lineup of medical pros ready to tackle your menopause blues. They offer a detailed health profile—developed according to guidelines from the American College of Gynecology and the North American Menopause Society—and then connect you with a clinician who can prescribe medication or offer advice for symptoms based on what you need. Sure, it'll cost you a bit ($49 per month), but who can put a price on feeling like yourself again?
- **Midday:** This one's like the Swiss Army knife of menopause apps, with everything from symptom tracking to connecting with health professionals. They even let you hook up your Fitbit or Apple Watch to get

the inside scoop on your sleep and activity levels. Talk about high-tech menopause management. You can enjoy a complimentary three-month trial, followed by a subscription fee of $29.99 every three months or $78 for an annual subscription.

- **Caria:** Consider it your trusty sidekick through the menopause maze. Not only does it help you track symptoms, but it also offers behavioral health options like cognitive therapy. Because, let's face it, sometimes you just need a little mental TLC to get through those sleepless nights and mood swings. It also offers help from life coaches, dietitians, and fitness trainers. The app provides a no-cost subscription with essential features, as well as a premium option offering "unlimited expert-crafted programs" for $9.99 per month or $49.99 annually. (Atkins, 2023)

So, why suffer in silence when you can have these apps in your corner, cheering you on through the menopause marathon? Give them a whirl, and let the journey to symptom relief begin.

Telehealth and Virtual Consultations

Now, picture this: You're cozied up on your couch with a cup of tea, maybe some dark chocolate (because, let's be real, chocolate is always a good idea), and you're chatting away with your healthcare professional through your laptop or smartphone. That's telehealth in action, sister.

Think about the convenience. No more rushing through traffic or sitting in sterile waiting rooms. With telehealth, you can get expert advice, learn about the latest treatments, and feel supported—all without changing out of your comfy pajamas. It's like having your own personal health guru right in your living room.

But here's the scoop: While telehealth is super handy, it's not a magic cure-all. Sure, it's fantastic for discussing symptoms, getting guidance, and feeling heard. Your doctor already knows you like the back of their hand, thanks to your shared health history and data, but hey, not every issue can be solved in this manner.

Take vaginal dryness, for instance. It's no joke, and it can have various causes. Menopause might be the culprit, but it's not the only suspect in town. Sometimes, you need a physical exam to rule out other sneaky troublemakers.

So, while telehealth is fantastic on this journey, remember to keep it real. Sometimes, that means showing up in person. Bottom line? Embrace the telehealth revolution—it's a game-changer for menopause warriors like us. But also know when it's time to put on real shoes and head to the doctor's office.

Educational Resources and Webinars

While we were busy conquering the world, nobody handed us a manual for this wild ride. By 2030, there will be over 1.2 billion of us negotiating the menopausal maze, with a cool 47 million newbies joining every year (Weiss, 2022). Talk about a power surge!

We need to start conversations earlier than we might think, around 35 or 40. Why? Well, because menopausal symptoms can kick in six to ten years before your last period.

Webinars and resources are your secret weapons for tackling menopause like a queen. Think of them as your virtual girl squad, cheering you on and dishing out the wisdom.

Visit Menopause at Work: Asia Pacific. There, you will find four amazing workshops surrounding mental health, your career, well-being, and self-care while transitioning through menopause.

Throughout this chapter, we've emphasized the vital role of building a support network and understanding the emotional side of menopause. It's crystal clear that having social and emotional support can truly make a difference in our lives during this journey. As we move forward, we'll delve into the significance of nurturing our mental well-being, exploring mindfulness practices and strategies for building resilience to ensure a well-rounded menopausal journey.

Chapter 6 Menopause Management Quiz: Unlocking Your Support Squad

Ready to assess your current support system and discover new tools for navigating menopause? Buckle up, goddesses! This light-hearted quiz will guide you through your inner circle and explore professional support options to create a powerful network for your journey.

Circle the answer that best reflects your current situation:

1. How often do you connect with other women about menopause?

- (a) We have regular "menopause mastermind" meetings or participate in online communities! (Often)
- (b) We chat occasionally, but it's not an ongoing thing. (Sometimes)
- (c) I mostly keep it to myself. (Rarely)

2. When you're feeling overwhelmed by menopause symptoms, do you have someone to vent to and receive understanding?

- (a) Absolutely! My support system is my rock, including friends, family, and even professionals. (Often)
- (b) Occasionally, but I feel like I'm burdening them. (Sometimes)
- (c) Not really, I try to manage it alone. (Rarely)

3. Have you considered seeking professional support from a therapist or counselor specializing in menopause?

- (a) Yes, and it's been incredibly helpful. (Often)
- (b) I'm curious, but haven't taken the plunge yet. (Sometimes)
- (c) Not really my preference, I prefer informal support. (Rarely)

4. Do you feel comfortable setting boundaries with loved ones about your needs and limitations during menopause?

- (a) I'm a boundary queen, my needs are always met. (Often)
- (b) I'm working on it, but it can be tricky. (Sometimes)
- (c) Boundaries? Isn't that just being demanding? (Rarely)

5. How often do you engage in shared activities with friends or family that bring joy and laughter?

- (a) We're constantly planning fun adventures, even if they're menopause-focused. (Often)
- (b) We get together occasionally, but activities aren't always menopause-focused. (Sometimes)

- (c) Most of my time is dedicated to managing symptoms. (Rarely)

6. Have you explored technology-based resources like menopause tracking apps, online forums, or telehealth consultations?

- (a) I'm a tech-savvy goddess, I use all the tools. (Often)
- (b) I've heard about them, but haven't used them yet. (Sometimes)
- (c) Not really my thing, I prefer traditional support methods. (Rarely)

Tally your answers:

- **Mostly (a)s:** You're a support system superhero! You have a strong network, utilize professional resources, and embrace technology. Keep fostering those connections and exploring new tools.
- **Mostly (b)s:** You're on the right track. Consider expanding your support network, connecting with a therapist, and exploring technology-based resources. Chapter 6 offers tips on navigating communication, setting boundaries, and finding valuable resources.
- **Mostly (c)s:** Remember, goddess, you don't have to go through this alone. Chapter 6 can help you build a supportive community, explore professional options, and leverage technology to navigate your journey. It's time to prioritize your well-being.

Remember: Building a strong support system with both personal connections and professional expertise is crucial for a smoother and more enriching menopause journey. Embrace the power of connection, empower yourself with the tools in Chapter 6, and remember, you're not alone.

Disclaimer: This quiz is intended for informational purposes only and should not be a substitute for professional medical advice. Always consult with a healthcare professional for personalized guidance.

NOTES:

_____

_____

_____

_____

_____

_____

_____

_____

_____

_____

_____

_____

_____

_____

_____

Chapter 7

Staying Balanced—Menopause and Mental Well-being

S tatistics show that a staggering 73% of women are navigating menopausal challenges without proper treatment. This includes grappling with issues like hot flashes (16%), weight gain (15%), difficulties with sleep (14%), and night sweats (14%), among others (Gordon, 2021). If this scenario resonates with you, know that you're not alone. In this chapter, embark on a journey to equip yourself with the mental fortitude and techniques needed to not only weather the storm but emerge stronger, more balanced, and mentally resilient. Discover empowering strategies to enhance your mental well-being during menopause.

Recognizing Signs of Depression

Let's debunk a myth: menopause isn't just about brain fog and erupting chin hair. Nope, it's a whole package deal that can come with its fair share of emotional twists and turns. One of those twists? Depression.

Now, how do we spot this unwelcome guest? Well, it's not always as obvious as you might think. Sure, we all have those days when we feel a bit down in the dumps, but when those blue moods start camping out for weeks on end, it might be time to pay closer attention.

Here are a few signs to watch out for:

- **Mood swings on steroids:** We're talking about mood swings that make pre-menstrual syndrome look like a walk in the park. If you find yourself bouncing between feeling on top of the world one minute and down in the dumps the next, it might be more than just your typical hormonal plunge.
- **Sleeping patterns gone haywire:** You used to be the queen of Snooze Ville, but now it feels like you're starring in your own late-night infomercials. If you're struggling to catch those Z's or finding yourself waking up at ungodly hours, depression might be lurking in the shadows.
- **Lost interest in things you once loved:** Remember that pottery class you used to adore? Or the book club you couldn't get enough of? If those once-beloved activities now feel like a job, it could be a sign that depression is crashing the party.
- **Constant fatigue:** We're not just talking about feeling a bit tired after a long day. This is the kind of fatigue that makes getting out of bed feel like scaling Mount Everest. When the thought of taking a shower makes you want to take a nap, If you find yourself constantly drained, it might be worth chatting with your doctor.
- **Changes in appetite:** Suddenly craving nothing but carbs or couldn't care less about food? Extreme changes

in appetite, whether it's overeating or barely touching your plate, can be another clue that something's amiss. (Payne, 2024)

Now, here's the good news: recognizing the signs is the first step toward kicking depression to the curb. So, what's next? Well, it's time to call in the reinforcements.

First, you should schedule an appointment with your doctor. Seriously, don't be shy about chatting with them about what's going on. They're armed with all sorts of tools to help you, whether it's therapy, medication, or a combination of both.

But hey, let's not forget about the power of good old-fashioned self-care. Yep, we're talking bubble baths, long walks in nature, and curling up with a good book. Whatever floats your boat and soothes your soul, make time for it.

And don't forget your support system. Whether it's your partner, your besties, or your furry friends, surround yourself with love and support. Because let's face it, life's too short to go it alone.

Anxiety in Menopause

It's totally normal to feel a bit jittery or on edge during menopause. Hormones are doing their funky dance, life is throwing its curveballs, and sleep seems to be playing hard to get —no wonder anxiety decides to join the fun. In fact, a bunch of Brazilian researchers found that over half of women aged 45 to 55 going through perimenopause experienced some level of anxiety (Railton, 2023). You're not alone in this boat.

Hormones can really stir the pot when they start fluctuating. Estrogen, in particular, seems to have a knack for triggering anxiety when it's playing hide-and-seek in your body (Railton,

2023). But hey, we're not letting those hormones have the upper hand—we have strategies.

Speaking of strategies, here's the lowdown on how to tackle anxiety head-on:

- **Get moving:** Yep, exercise can do wonders for your mental well-being. So, lace up those sneakers and bust a move—whether it's a brisk walk, a Pilates session, or dancing in your living room, find what moves your soul and go for it. Can't make yourself go it alone? Try volunteering at the local animal shelter to walk dogs. Doing something nice for others feels great and happiness is contagious.
- **Watch your caffeine and alcohol intake:** While they might seem like good companions during stressful times, they can actually amp up your anxiety levels. So, maybe swap that third cup of coffee for a soothing herbal tea and dial back on the wine nights.
- **Try acupuncture:** It's not just for poking fun—it can actually help ease anxiety symptoms. Plus, it's a great excuse for a little self-care session.
- **Sleep:** I know it can be elusive during menopause, but making it a priority can work wonders for your anxiety levels. Create a cozy bedtime routine, banish screens from the bedroom, and embrace the power of a good night's sleep.
- **Lean on your support system:** Support groups are like a warm hug for your soul. Whether it's a bunch of girlfriends, an online community, or a therapy group, having people who get what you're going through can be incredibly comforting. (Railton, 2023)

And finally, don't forget to treat yourself like the queen you are. Take time for activities that nourish your spirit. Maybe you like digging in your garden or getting lost in a good book? Remember, you have the power to turn those anxious moments into opportunities for growth and self-care. Remember, your mental health is the most important. Don't hesitate to reach out to your healthcare team and discuss options with them as well.

Cognitive Function and Brain Health

Brain Fog and Memory Lapses

Ever find yourself frantically searching for your phone, only to realize it's been in your hand the whole time? Or maybe you've wandered into a room and completely forgotten why you went in there in the first place? Welcome to the world of brain fog, a common symptom experienced by up to two-thirds of women going through menopause (*How to Combat Menopausal Brain Fog*, 2022).

Let's explore some strategies for combating this foggy phenomenon. While "brain fog" isn't a clinical term, it's the relatable way many people describe changes in memory and thinking. According to the Australasian Menopause Society, menopausal brain fog can show up as difficulty focusing, feeling easily distracted, misplacing items, and experiencing time slips (*How to Combat Menopausal Brain Fog*, 2022).

Strategies for Improving Concentration

It almost begins to feel like a daily occurrence, wondering where you left your glasses or what time your appointment is. Yep, we've all been there and done that. There are ways to tame the unruly beast of menopausal mental fog. Let's talk lifestyle tweaks:

- **Get moving:** Exercise isn't just for youngsters; it's a magic potion for the mind, too. Aim for at least 30 minutes of exercise most days. Get that blood pumping to the brain and those endorphins flowing.
- **Prioritize sleep:** Menopause can play havoc with our sleep patterns, but don't let it win. Stick to a regular sleep schedule, create a relaxing bedtime routine, and banish those screens from the bedroom. Your brain will thank you for it.
- **Stress less:** Easier said than done, right? But finding ways to manage stress can do wonders for your concentration. Whether it's meditation, deep breathing exercises, or simply taking time for yourself to indulge in a hobby, make stress relief a priority.
- **Brain games:** Keep that gray matter on its toes with brain-teasing activities. Crossword puzzles, Sudoku, or even learning a new language can help sharpen your focus and memory.
- **Stay social**: Surround yourself with your support system and share a laugh or two. Socializing not only boosts mood but also stimulates your brain and keeps it firing on all cylinders.
- **Just say no:** Illicit substances, excessive booze, and smoking are like those shady characters trying to crash your party— show them the door and keep the good vibes rolling, shall we?
- **Get organized:** Give your days some structure and bid adieu to anxiety. And if you're prone to forgetting things faster than you can say, "Where are my keys?" let technology be your wingman with calendars and

reminders—because who needs forgetfulness cramping their style?

- **Seek support**: Don't be afraid to reach out for help if you're struggling. Whether it's talking to a friend, joining a support group, or seeking professional advice, there's strength in seeking support. (*How to Combat Menopausal Brain Fog*, 2022)

Brain-Boosting Activities and Games

We now understand that memory issues during menopause are often linked to the drop in estrogen. It plays a big role in language skills, mood, attention, and memory, so when this hormone decreases, it can mess with our brainpower. Now, the big question is, how do we tackle this? Studies have shown that engaging in 20 minutes daily of brain-boosting games can make a huge difference (Dunleavy, 2022).

- **Sudoku showdown:** Channel your inner mathlete and dive into the world of Sudoku puzzles. These number-filled grids aren't just fun—they're like a mental workout for your brain. Plus, there's something oddly satisfying about filling in those little squares with the right numbers. It's like cracking a secret code, one square at a time. So grab a pencil, get those neurons firing, and conquer those Sudokus like the brainiac you are.
- **Crossword crusade:** Let's face it—crossword puzzles are the original brain game. They're challenging, they're entertaining, and they make you feel like a linguistic genius when you finally fill in that last word. Plus, they're a sneaky way to expand your vocabulary without even trying. So grab a cup of coffee, cozy up with a

crossword, and get ready to flex those word-wrangling muscles. Who knows? You might just discover your inner crossword champion.

- **Memory match-up:** Remember playing Memory as a kid? Well, guess what—it's not just for the young kids. Memory games are a fantastic way to keep your cognitive skills sharp and your memory in tip-top shape. Plus, they're a blast to play, whether you're flying solo or challenging a friend. So, dust off those old cards, shuffle them up and get ready to test your memory prowess.

Nutritional Support for Cognitive Health

One of the most powerful tools in your arsenal? Nutrition. Yep, what you put on your plate can have a major impact on your cognitive health and overall mood. So, let's rehash some tasty tips:

- **Omega-3 fatty acids:** These bad boys are brain fuel. Studies have shown that omega-3s can help reduce symptoms of depression and support overall cognitive function. Load up on oily fish like salmon, walnuts, chia seeds, and flaxseeds to give your brain the boost it deserves.
- **B vitamins:** Say hello to your new best friends: The family of B vitamins. B1, B2, B3, B5, B6, B7, B9, and B12. Vitaly important to health, these little gems play a crucial role in brain health and can help ease symptoms of anxiety and depression. Load up on leafy greens, whole grains, eggs, and lean meats to get your daily B vitamin fix.
- **Antioxidants:** Think of antioxidants as your body's personal bodyguards, protecting your brain from

inflammation and oxidative stress. Load up on colorful fruits and veggies like berries, kale, and sweet potatoes to give your brain the anti-oxidant boost it craves.

- **Protein:** Don't skimp on the protein, ladies. Protein-rich foods contain amino acids that help regulate your mood and keep your brain firing on all cylinders. Opt for lean sources like fish, chicken, tofu, beans, and lentils to keep your mental game strong. (Yeager, 2022a)

And hey, just in case you forgot, hydrate, hydrate, hydrate. I can't say it too many times. Drinking plenty of water is crucial for cognitive function and overall well-being. Grab that water bottle and sip your way to mental clarity.

Self Care and Relaxation

Let's discuss the significance of self-care and relaxation during menopause. Right now, your hormones are all over the place, your body feels unsettled, and your mood is as unpredictable as the spring weather. Does this sound familiar? However, amid the chaos, there is a source of hope: self-care. It serves as a rejuvenating elixir that nurtures your spirit, calms your soul, and guides your hormones in a positive direction.

Now, I know what you're thinking. "But I barely have time to finish a cup of coffee, let alone indulge in self-care rituals." Trust me, I hear you loud and clear. But here's the thing: prioritizing yourself isn't selfish; it's survival. So, let's get creative with our relaxation techniques, shall we?

Relaxation Techniques

Alright, ladies, let's talk about relaxation during menopause. It's all about getting cozy with your breathing patterns. See, your emotions like to mess with your breathing. Anxious? You might catch yourself holding your breath, sounding like a chipmunk on helium. Feeling blue? You might find yourself sighing like you're auditioning for a dramatic movie role.

I've got some relaxation exercises that'll have you feeling fabulous in no time. Find yourself a quiet spot, get comfy, and kick those distracting thoughts to the curb:

- **Rhythmic breathing:** If you're huffing and puffing like you just sprinted a marathon, slow it down. Take deep, slow breaths. Count to five as you inhale, and count to five as you exhale. Feel your body chillaxing with each exhale. Ahh, feels good, right?
- **Deep breathing:** Imagine a spot right below your belly button. Breathe into it, filling up your belly like a balloon. Then, let it out slowly. Feel that tension melting away with each exhale. It's like your own personal deflate mode.
- **Visualized breathing:** Close your eyes and let your imagination run wild. Picture relaxation flowing into your body and stress flowing out. Breathe deeply and visualize each breath, bringing in relaxation and kicking out tension.
- **Progressive muscle relaxation:** Take a mental inventory of your body and where it's holding onto tension. Loosen up those tight spots, roll your head and shoulders, and let every muscle go limp. Think of something pleasant for a second, take a deep

breath, and feel that sweet, sweet relaxation wash over you.

- **Relax to music:** Cue up your favorite tunes and let the music work its magic. Whether it's uplifting beats or soothing melodies, let the music serenade you into a state of blissful calm.
- **Mental imagery relaxation:** Time to take a mental vacation. Picture yourself in your happy place, far away from stress and worries. And hey, while you're at it, flip the script on those negative thoughts with some positive affirmations. Repeat after me: "I've got this. I'm a powerhouse. Nothing can bring me down!" (WebMD Editorial Contributors, 2023b)

Creating a Personal Sanctuary

I want you to imagine a space you can disappear into whenever you need a break from the chaos of life. A sanctuary that's all about YOU, tailored to your tastes and needs. So, let's dive into creating this haven of tranquility, shall we?

- **Cozy comforts:** Start by surrounding yourself with things that bring you joy. Think soft blankets, plush pillows, and maybe even a snuggly pet if you have one. Having a cozy corner to curl up in can work wonders for your mental well-being.
- **Calming colors:** Choose colors that soothe your soul. Whether it's calming blues, earthy greens, or warm neutrals, pick hues that make you feel relaxed and at peace. Consider painting the walls or adding accents like curtains or throw rugs in your chosen palette.
- **Natural elements:** Bring a touch of nature indoors to reconnect with the earth's grounding energy.

Incorporate houseplants, seashells, or smooth stones into your sanctuary for a refreshing vibe.

- **Mindful moments:** Dedicate a space for mindfulness practices like meditation or yoga. It doesn't have to be big—even a small corner with a cushion or yoga mat will do. This is your sacred spot to breathe, stretch, and center yourself.
- **Sensory delights:** Engage your senses with soothing scents, calming sounds, and tactile textures. Consider adding essential oil diffusers, sound machines, or a fuzzy rug underfoot to enhance your sanctuary experience.
- **Personal touches:** Don't forget to infuse your sanctuary with personal touches that reflect your passions and interests. Whether it's framed photos of loved ones, inspirational quotes, favorite books, or artwork that speaks to your soul, surround yourself with reminders of what matters most to you.

Remember, your sanctuary is all about creating a space where you can recharge and find peace amidst the storm of menopause. So, get creative, have fun, and make it uniquely yours. You deserve a little oasis of calm in this crazy world.

Hobbies and Leisure Activities

Engaging in activities you love isn't just about passing the time; it's about feeding your soul and giving your mental health the care it deserves. Whether it's painting, gardening, dancing like nobody's watching, or solving Sudoku puzzles, hobbies have this magical power to transport you to a place where menopause symptoms are mere background noise.

Think about it: when was the last time you lost yourself in something you're passionate about? Remember that feeling of pure bliss, where time seemed to stand still, and your worries melted away like ice cream on a hot summer day? That, my friend, is the power of hobbies.

Engaging in activities you enjoy isn't just about escapism; it's also about empowerment. It's about reminding yourself that you're more than just a vessel for hormones gone haywire. You're a force to be reckoned with, capable of conquering anything that comes your way, power surges be damned.

So, here's the deal: make a date with yourself and your favorite hobby. Schedule it in like you would a doctor's appointment. Prioritize your mental well-being like the goddess that you are because you deserve it.

And hey, if you're not sure where to start, don't sweat it. Try something new, take a leap of faith, and see where it takes you. The world is your oyster, and menopause is just another adventure waiting to be conquered.

Building Resilience and Empowerment

Resilience refers to the ability to swiftly recover from challenges. (Kelly, 2016). Does menopause qualify? Absolutely!

We aren't born with resilience; it is a learned behavior. Let's look at how to build it:

- **Make connections:** Accepting assistance and encouragement from those who genuinely care about you and are willing to listen can enhance resilience.
- **Find the silver lining:** Look ahead to envision a slightly brighter tomorrow.

- **Accept that change is normal:** Accepting that there will always be things beyond our control and cannot be changed can help you focus on the things you can control.
- **Set achievable goals:** Engage in regular activities that propel you toward a new goal. If you aim to improve your eating habits, what steps can you take today to initiate that change?
- **Nurture a positive view of yourself:** Develop self-confidence and trust your instincts to enhance resilience.
- **Keep perspective:** Consider the stressful situation within a broader context and maintain a long-term perspective. Menopause may feel never-ending, but it is not permanent.
- **Be hopeful:** Instead of dwelling on what you've lost, try visualizing what you still have and will gain.
- **Take care of yourself:** Pay close attention to your own needs and emotions. Participate in activities that bring you joy and promote relaxation. (Kelly, 2016)

Picture this: you're the CEO of your own life, and menopause is just an interloper trying to mess with your agenda. Sure, it might throw you off course now and then, but you've got the power to steer the ship. Embrace the changes, embrace the challenges, and, most importantly, embrace yourself. You're a force to be reckoned with, and menopause is just a temporary blip on the radar.

Setting goals for personal growth? Heck, yes, count us in. Whether it's finally taking that yoga class you've been considering, reigniting your passion for painting, or simply committing to self-care Sundays, now's the time to prioritize YOU. Menopause is the beginning of a new chapter filled with endless possibilities.

So go ahead, dream big, set those goals, and watch yourself blossom like never before.

Throughout your menopausal journey, your mental well-being needs to be your first priority. It sets the stage for a positive post-menopausal phase.

You are about to step into the future, moving away from menopause and into post-menopause with all its opportunities and challenges.

Get ready to step into the next chapter, the final part of our WELLNESS framework. We will focus on navigating post-menopause with insights into physical health, lifestyle adjust-ments, and emotional well-being.

Chapter 7 Menopause Management Quiz: Nurturing Your Mind & Body

Ready to assess your current strategies for self-care, relaxation, and building resilience during menopause? Buckle up, goddess. This quiz will guide you through your self-love practices, covering key areas like stress management, relaxation techniques, and setting intentions for personal growth. Remember, a lighthearted approach is key!

Instructions:

For each statement, select the option that best reflects your current habits:

1. Self-care is a necessity, not a luxury.

- I prioritize self-care rituals like baths, journaling, or spending time in nature to nourish my mind and body. (Often)

- I occasionally indulge in self-care, but it doesn't always make it to the top of my to-do list. (Sometimes)
- I struggle to prioritize myself and often feel guilty taking time for self-care. (Rarely)

2. When stress tries to crash your party, do you have relaxation techniques in your arsenal?

- I actively manage stress through techniques like deep breathing, meditation, relaxing walks or listening to calming music. (Often)
- I know some relaxation techniques, but I don't use them consistently when stressed. (Sometimes)
- Stress often takes control, and I haven't explored effective ways to manage it. (Rarely)

3. The idea of creating a personal sanctuary is a necessity not just a dream.

- I've created a cozy haven filled with things I love, offering a space for peace and relaxation. (Often)
- I haven't dedicated a specific space for self-care, but I find pockets of calmness throughout my home. (Sometimes)
- My living environment doesn't promote relaxation, and I haven't prioritized creating a dedicated sanctuary. (Rarely)

4. Hobbies and leisure activities are joyful pursuits not just an afterthought.

- I schedule time for activities I truly enjoy, like painting, dancing, or reading, to nourish my soul. (Often)

- I have hobbies, but they often fall by the wayside due to other demands. (Sometimes)
- Finding time for activities I enjoy feels impossible, and I rarely engage in anything purely recreational. (Rarely)

5. When faced with challenges, do you bounce back with resilience or feel easily overwhelmed?

- I practice self-compassion, seek support when needed, and maintain a positive outlook even during difficult times. (Often)
- I sometimes struggle with setbacks but try to find the silver lining and move forward. (Sometimes)
- Challenges often leave me feeling defeated and discouraged, and I have difficulty coping with setbacks. (Rarely)

6. Setting personal goals feels daunting, especially during menopause.

- I set achievable goals for personal growth and celebrate my progress along the way. (Often)
- I occasionally set goals but struggle with consistency and motivation, especially during challenging times. (Sometimes)
- Setting goals feels overwhelming, and I haven't focused on personal growth recently. (Rarely)

Tally up your score using this system:

- **Often (3 points)**
- **Sometimes (2 points)**
- **Rarely (1 point)**

Once you've got your tally, check it against this:

- **15-18 points:** You're a self-care superhero. You prioritize your well-being and actively manage challenges with effective strategies. Keep rocking it!
- **10–15 points:** You're on the right track. Consider incorporating new self-care practices from the aforementioned tips and explore resources like meditation apps or support groups. Chapter 7 offers in-depth guidance.
- **0–9 points:** Remember, goddess, you deserve to prioritize your well-being. Chapter 7 provides a roadmap for building a self-care toolkit, exploring relaxation techniques, and cultivating resilience. Don't hesitate to reach out for support and remember, you've got this!

Disclaimer: This quiz is intended for informational purposes only and should not be a substitute for professional medical advice. Always consult with a healthcare professional for personalized guidance.

NOTES:

_____

_____

_____

_____

_____

_____

_____

_____

_____

_____

_____

_____

_____

_____

_____

_____

_____

_____

_____

_____

_____

_____

_____

_____

_____

_____

_____

Chapter 8

Stepping into the Future—Navigating Post-Menopause

> " *Diversity makes for a rich tapestry, and you must understand that all the threads of the tapestry are equal in value, no matter their color.*
>
> — *Maya Angelou*

Step boldly into the future of post-menopause, where the path is paved with opportunities, and the tapestry of life unfolds in vibrant colors. Each thread of your life holds immense value, and the post-menopausal phase is no exception. Prepare to navigate post-menopause with confidence, embracing wisdom and ensuring long-term health.

Future Focused Health: Beyond Menopause

Alright, ladies, let's talk about crossing that finish line into the post-menopausal phase.

Transitioning into the Post-Menopausal Phase

You've now officially bid farewell to Aunt Flo for 12 months straight—yep, that's the signal that post-menopause has welcomed you with open arms. Now, statistically speaking, this milestone typically hits around age 51, give or take a few years. So, if you find yourself in the 45 to 55 age group, you're right on track for this grand entrance into the post-menopausal club (*Post-menopause*, 2021).

But hey, once you're in, you're in for the long haul—post-menopause is your new forever home. Your hormone levels have diminished, bidding adieu to estrogen and progesterone. And guess what? No more surprise monthly visits from Mother Nature because your ovaries have called it quits on releasing eggs. You are officially off the hook for pregnancy scares—cheers to that.

Now, let's talk about the infamous hot flashes, or power surges, as I like to call them. Oh, they're still lurking around post-menopause, fueled by those decreased estrogen levels. Rest assured, they won't be as frequent. It's like your body's way of keeping you on your toes, even when you least expect it. While post-menopause may come with its quirks, it's also a time of newfound freedom and empowerment.

Longevity and Aging Gracefully

Your ovaries are like time travelers, sprinting into the future while the rest of your body plays catch-up.From birth, they're packing millions of follicles, each one holding the promise of future eggs. But by the time you hit 51, the average age of menopause in the U.S., those follicles are as scarce as a parking spot at your favorite restaurant on Valentine's Day (Mullin, 2023).

Now, here's where it gets interesting. While humans (and some whales) might be the only species throwing menopause parties, it doesn't mean we're doomed to a life of symptoms. Sure, the loss of hormones can throw us a few curveballs—think brittle bones, slower metabolism, and a higher risk of various health issues (Mullin, 2023)—but, believe it or not, other than doing our best to manage the results of having fewer hormones, science is working on how to make those ovaries stick around just a bit longer, which might be the secret sauce to longevity and aging with grace. Studies show that delaying menopause could up your chances of hitting that coveted age of 90. And get this: transplanting young ovaries into older mice actually made them live 40% longer (Mullin, 2023). Talk about the fountain of youth!

While we're not quite there yet in the realm of human trials hey, progress is progress, right? The good news is that the scientific community is finally giving female reproductive aging the attention it deserves. So, who knows? Maybe we'll crack this code sooner than we think.

In the meantime, let's focus on what we can control: staying active, eating well, and embracing the journey with a healthy dose of humor. After all, laughter is the best medicine, especially when you're dealing with a time-traveling ovary or two.

A Time to Reflect on Your Health

Low estrogen levels aren't just a numbers game—they're behind some serious health shakedowns as we age. We're talking osteoporosis (those fragile bones are no joke) and heart disease to name two. Did you know more women die from heart disease than breast cancer (Spencer, n.d.)? Estrogen actually protects your heart, and its disappearance post-menopause? Well, let's just say it's like leaving a turtle without its shell.

But hold up, before you start building a fortress of pillows around yourself, know this: you've got more control than you think. Lifestyle changes are your trusty sidekick in this hormonal detective story. As we've discussed, ditching the cigarettes, keeping the alcohol in check, shedding those extra pounds, and giving your body the love it deserves with some good old-fashioned exercise —these are your weapons for continued health.

Now, let's talk bones—because who doesn't want to stay sturdy and strong? Osteoporosis steals bone strength as we age, making us more prone to fractures. It's especially tricky for women after menopause, who can lose up to 20% of their bone density in just a few years. Weight-bearing exercises are the antidote to osteoporosis, keeping those bones fortified and ready to take on the world (Spencer, n.d.).

During post-menopause, you may notice your bladder feeling a bit cranky, too, thanks to the estrogen disappearing act. It's like a balloon that's lost its bounce, causing some unwanted squeezes and discomfort. Your doctor's heard it all before, so don't be shy about asking for help because there are medications and surgery that can help (Spencer, n.d.).

And let's not forget about your lady bits—they deserve special care too. Vaginal dryness and atrophy are common in post-menopause, but here's the good news: most of these symptoms are as treatable. So, don't suffer in silence—reach out for help (Spencer, n.d.).

Advanced Preventive Health Measures

Let's talk about what's on the horizon for your health beyond this phase of life.

So, here's the deal: when it comes to post-menopause, there's a bit of a gap in how we approach clinical care, policy, and education for both us women and providers. It's like we've hit a speed bump on the road to understanding and managing this transition effectively.

You see, both patients and doctors alike aren't fully clued in on what to expect after menopause. This lack of understanding can lead to delays in recognizing the post-menopausal transition and tackling those accompanying symptoms head-on.

To turn things around and improve the quality of life for all of us wonderful women, we need changes to the system. First off, let's standardize how we prepare for menopause. To date, amazingly enough, menopause isn't even covered in the regular medical school curriculum. This needs to change. We need to educate both women and our healthcare providers so we know what's coming and how to handle it (Aninye et al., 2021).

We also need to shake things up on the policy front. There are regulatory hurdles that can make accessing care a real headache.

And don't even get me started on the lack of research funding for menopause-related studies. The National Institutes of Health Research Portfolio Online Reporting Tools system assists users in keeping track of annual research funding for different health conditions. Surprisingly, even though all women will experience menopause, it's not even listed as one of the 292 topics, unlike infertility or pregnancy. In 2019, only 28 research projects included the term menopause, yet 300 included pregnancy. This shows the need for better prioritization of federal investment in menopause research to fill those knowledge gaps in the field (Aninye et al., 2021).

And here's a little secret: menopause isn't a disease—it's just another chapter in the incredible journey of womanhood. So, we need to continue on the path of ditching the stigma and embracing it for what it is: a natural part of life.

To sum it all up, we're on a mission to empower you with knowledge, support, and research. Here's to embracing the future with open arms.

Embracing New Horizons

In earlier generations, women underwent menopause at a later age and had shorter lifespans compared to the present day. Now, our post-menopausal phase will make up 40% of our entire lifespan (Spencer, n.d.).

Menopause is like a life evaluation package deal. It's the perfect time to take stock of our physical and mental well-being, happiness, and priorities and then craft a plan for an awesome new chapter. For many women, bidding farewell to menstruation feels liberating, and as their symptoms subside, they find a renewed zest for life.

Rediscovering Personal Interests and Passions

This is a chance to shake things up, rewrite the script, and rediscover the fabulousness that is you.

Think of it as a midlife metamorphosis. You're shedding the skin of your reproductive years and emerging as a butterfly of wisdom, experience, and, yes, maybe a few stray gray hairs.

Sure, there are changes happening, but amid all that, there's an invitation to dive deep into your passions, interests, and dreams— the ones that may have taken a backseat to life's hustle and bustle.

Menopause is a golden opportunity to dust off those forgotten hobbies, reignite those old flames of passion, and chase after the things that light you up inside.

So, whether it's picking up that paintbrush you abandoned years ago, dusting off your camera, or finally taking that cooking class you've been eyeing, embrace it all with open arms.

This is your time to shine. So, go ahead, lean into the change, and let's make menopause the most fabulous chapter yet.

Pursuing New Goals and Aspirations

Rita's Story

Throughout my life, I always believed I took great care of myself. I married my best friend, we had three amazing children, and they blessed us with five grandchildren. I had a job that helped me provide for my family and a home I loved. My friends were always there to support and love me; what more could a girl ask for, right?

When menopause shook up my world, I fell apart. I started to question everything. Was I really happy? Did I truly feel content? Was this all life had to offer? After sitting in my therapist's office once a week for a solid year, it all became clear.

I had spent the last 35 years providing for those I loved. I was a picture perfect wife, mother, friend, daughter, sister, coworker, and well... you get the picture. I lost my sense of self in all of that. At no point did I check in with myself and ask if I was okay. I failed to make sure I was getting what I needed.

I realized my job did offer financial security, but it left me flat. I punched in numbers all day and felt numb while I sat there staring at a computer screen. It didn't ignite a passion in my soul, and I was missing that. I was an avid photographer before having my children, and somewhere along the line, I told myself I had no time for that.

I sat down with my husband and told him I needed more in my life. Realistically, I could live another 35 to 40 years, and I wanted them to have meaning. He was supportive and asked questions. Within a month, I quit my job and went back to school. I fine-tuned my photography skills and opened my own business.
I now spend my days taking pictures of giggling children, and it fills my heart. I make a point to check in with myself regularly. Am I happy, am I content, and is there anything else I want to try? I highly suggest others do the same.

Now, I know it's easy to get caught up in the whirlwind of change, but let's focus on the bright side, shall we? It's time to dust off those dreams and let them shine. Need some inspiration? Here are ten goals and aspirations to get your mojo flowing:

- **Learn something new:** Have you always wanted to play the piano or guitar or learn to speak Italian? Go for it with gusto.
- **Travel:** Pack your bags and hit the road—exploring new places and cultures is food for the soul.
- **Start a passion project:** Whether it's writing that novel or launching a business, channel your creativity into something you love.
- **Go back to school:** Inspired by Rita's story? Have you always wished you pursued your education in a different direction? Why not now? You are never too old to learn.
- **Volunteer:** Making a difference in your community is not only rewarding but also a great way to connect with like-minded souls.
- **Embrace your inner chef:** It's time to whip up those gourmet dishes you've been drooling over on Pinterest.
- **Rediscover romance:** Whether it's with a partner or yourself, prioritize pleasure and intimacy. Light those

candles, book a weekend away.
- **Master mindfulness:** Practice meditation or journaling to quiet the mind and find inner peace.
- **Invest in relationships:** Strengthen bonds with friends and family—it's all about love and laughter.
- **Set boundaries:** Say goodbye to people-pleasing and hello to honoring your own needs and desires.

Advancing Personal Development

This is a crucial moment for you. Instead of focusing only on the difficulties, menopause can be seen as a chance to grow personally and professionally. Think of it as a way to discover more about yourself and feel more powerful, helping you to accept and strengthen your inner resilience.

What to Expect from Your Employer

The menopause journey might lead you to rethink your career goals and priorities. And guess what? That's totally okay. Some of us might decide it's time for a major career shift or to dial back on our work responsibilities a bit. And yeah, the challenges of menopause can sometimes make climbing that career ladder feel like scaling Everest in stilettos. Ageism and biases? Yep, they're real. We should be demanding our employers step up to the plate and make a real difference.

Picture this: tailored development programs, inclusive leadership, transparent evaluations—these are the tools that can help smash through those glass ceilings. But hey, communication is key. Don't be afraid to chat with your bosses about what you need. And yes, I get it: revealing your menopausal status might feel like handing over a vulnerability pass. But here's the thing: you deserve support, not stigma.

Organizations need to start talking openly about menopause, educating everyone, and putting policies in place to support women like us. Because, let's face it, a supportive work culture isn't just a nice-to-have—it's a necessity.

And you? You're a force to be reckoned with. Embrace those strengths, seek out mentors, and grab hold of every chance for growth and development. Continuous learning? Check. Adapting like a boss? Double check. Your skills and experience are pure gold, and it's about time everyone recognized it.

Lifelong Learning and Skill Development

It's time to explore the topic of lifelong learning and skill development. Some might think, "Wait a minute, I'm already dealing with enough; why should I bother learning new things now?" Well, here's the tea: embracing lifelong learning is like giving your brain a spa day. It keeps those neurons firing, sharpens your cognitive skills, and reduces the risk of cognitive decline (*The Many Benefits*, n.d.). Who doesn't want to be a sharp-as-a-tack, quick-witted maven in their golden years?

Plus, let's not forget the thrill of mastering something new. Whether it's picking up a new language (Bonjour, French lover), diving into the wonderful world of coding, or becoming the local expert on generative AI there's a sense of accomplishment that comes with expanding our skill set. It's never too late to start. Did you know that around 41% of women aged 55–64 are enrolled in some form of education or training (Ferguson, 2016)?

Learning new skills isn't just about keeping our brains sharp. It's about reinventing ourselves, exploring passions we've put on the back burner, and embracing the badassery of stepping out of our comfort zones. So, why hesitate? Dive headfirst into that pottery class, dust off your camera or unleash your inner Picasso, and let's show the world that menopause isn't just about surviving; it's about thriving.

Exploring Creative Pursuits

Welcome to the wise woman's cycle, where the real fun begins. Your kids might be more independent now, your career settled, and your relationships a bit more predictable. Translation? You've got some breathing room, sister.

You finally have the time to dust off the dreams you tucked away ages ago. Remember that novel you started or that jewelry-making class you always wanted to take? It's time to reclaim those passions, my friend.

Some holistic people talk about a power surge in your chakras during menopause. Basically, all that energy that used to hang around your lady bits is now doing a happy dance up your spine, unlocking a newfound sense of intuition and creative zest for life. Pretty cool, right?

Ready to channel that inner goddess? Here are seven kick-ass ways to unleash your creativity:

1. Take a leisurely stroll and soak in the world around you. Feel the breeze on your skin, listen to the birds chirping, smell the roses (or the city air, depending on your locale). Let your senses guide you to your next masterpiece, whether it's a poem, a painting, or a killer Instagram post.
2. Break a sweat. Exercise isn't just for sculpting that body; it's a powerful stress-buster, too. Whether you're into

brisk walks or downward dogs, moving your body can be the ultimate form of self-expression.

3. Revisit your roots. Remember those hobbies you loved before life got crazy? Explore your family's genealogy, dust off that old sketchbook or crack open that half written novel hiding in your drawer. It's time to reignite those flames, baby.

4. Hit up your local library. They're not just for bookworms anymore. They are a social hub of activity. Find a local jewelry-making class or bust a move in an adult dance session. Who knows? You might discover a hidden talent for the tango.

5. Try a paint-and-sip class. Because who says creativity can't come with a side of vino? Let loose, paint outside the lines, and maybe make some new friends while you're at it.

6. Learn to knit like a boss. Not only will you impress your friends with your newfound skills, but studies say it's as soothing as a spa day (minus the hefty price tag) (James, 2017). At the same time you'll keep your hands busy (not snacking) and you'll end up with some beautiful throws, blankets, hats, (whatever) to gift.

7. Get wild in the kitchen. Whip up exotic dishes, raid your local farmers' market for inspiration, and let your taste buds go on an adventure. Then treat your friends.

Global Perspectives on Post-Menopause

It's like the ultimate plot twist: Western women seem to be taking the trophy for experiencing the most intense menopausal roller-coaster ride. But hold up, before we blame it all on biology, let's take a step back and look at the bigger picture of social and cultural factors at play.

In Western societies, we've got this funny little habit of treating older women like they're past their prime, right? It's like we've got a one-way ticket to the sidelines of society. But that's not the case everywhere else on this big blue marble we call earth. In some places, menopause is revered as a time of wisdom and empowerment.

American women are finally catching on. We're starting to realize that menopause isn't just about night sweats and mood swings; it's a freaking spiritual awakening, people! It's our metamorphosis from regular Janes into fierce Wonder Women.

Need proof? Just look around. More and more women over 50 are dominating the scene, whether it's strutting their stuff on the political stage or slaying it in the entertainment industry. Who said menopause was the end of the line? We're just getting started, baby.

Cultural Approaches to Aging and Menopause

Menopause in Japan

We're taking a trip to Japan, where menopause, or *konenki* as they call it, kicks in around the early 40s and hangs around until about 60. Now, they've got this whole different vibe about it. Instead of seeing it as the body going haywire, they view it as a time of renewal and regeneration (*Menopause in Different Cultures*, 2023). Beautiful, isn't it?

You see, the Japanese don't sweat the small stuff when it comes to menopause. And hey, maybe it's because of how they break down the word *konenki*. *Ko* for "renewal and regeneration," *nen* for "year," and *ki* for "season" or "energy." It's like a slow dance toward change, where bidding farewell to Aunt Flo is just one part of the journey (*Menopause in Different Cultures*, 2023).

Meanwhile, we Westerners are over here treating menopause like it's the kiss of death. Our term for it, "menopause," sounds like a bad Greek tragedy—*men* meaning "month" and *pausis* meaning "stop." (*Menopause in Different Cultures*, 2023).

The Japanese seem to have cracked the code on dodging menopausal mayhem. While we're grabbing a quick burger and fries, they're savoring soybeans and loading up on phytoestrogens and isoflavones. Is it the diet magic? Maybe. Is it their Zen-like approach to life? It is a good possibility. Either way, they're winning in the health department.

I'm talking about the longest life expectancy, minimal chronic issues, and a bone density that puts ours to shame. Oh, and did I mention their breast cancer rates? A mere fraction of ours. It's like they're playing a whole different game of health bingo (*Menopause in Different Cultures*, 2023).

So, what's their secret sauce? Well, it's a mix of diet, exercise, education, healthcare access, and a pinch of cultural mojo. Turns out, they've been into this whole preventive healthcare thing for ages.

Menopause for Mayan Women

Alright, let's bust some myths about the Mayans. Turns out, they're not just ancient history gathering dust in textbooks. Nope, they're still kicking it in rural Guatemala and parts of Mexico, shedding light on menopause like never before.

Scientists, armed with curiosity, ventured into these Mayan communities, aiming to uncover the secrets of menopause. And what do they find? A mixed bag of surprises. Some Mayan women breeze through menopause like a walk in the park, while others, well, they're not so lucky. It's like a menopausal roulette— you never know what you're gonna get (*Menopause in Different Cultures*, 2023).

Now, here's where it gets interesting. Despite the odds, these Mayan ladies seem to have cracked the code on dodging the dreaded osteoporosis monster. Yep, their estrogen levels dip, their bone density takes a hit, but fractures? Nah, not on their watch (*Menopause in Different Cultures*, 2023).

While we're tossing and turning in menopausal misery, these Mayan women are looking forward to it. Yeah, you heard me right. They're embracing this whole menopause thing like it's the best thing ever.

So, what's their secret? Well, it's a cocktail of natural herbs, a laid-back lifestyle, and a sprinkle of cultural attitudes. Oh, and let's not forget their newfound status as spiritual leaders post-menopause (*Menopause in Different Cultures*, 2023). It's like they're leveling up.

Connecting with International Menopause Communities

Sometimes, it's not just about the physical stuff. It's about finding your people, your support system, your squad who gets what you're going through. Luckily, we're living in an age where you can connect with like-minded women from across all cultures with just a few clicks. So, why not dip your toe into international menopause communities? Whether it's joining online forums, attending virtual support groups, or even planning a ladies' getaway with newfound friends, we can learn a great deal from each other about how to treat our symptoms and live a healthy life from one another. Seeing this entire menopausal journey through the eyes of others offers a huge benefit. There's strength in solidarity.

We covered a lot of important material in this final chapter. It was important to make sure we ended this amazing book on a positive note. We, as women transitioning through this phase, are often left feeling isolated, alone, and without answers or hope. This final chapter was hoped to show you that life after menopause can be amazing.

We discussed the importance of holistic wellness during post-menopause. Why it is crucial, now more than ever, to take care of your body and mind. This is the final step of the WELLNESS framework, achieving complete well-being.

I invite you to turn the page for a quick recap in the conclusion of this book. I promise a reflective and relatable wrap-up of the menopause journey and how you can be excited about your future with confidence, vitality, and empowerment.

Chapter 8 Menopause Management Quiz: A Guide to Post Menopausal Empowerment

This quiz guides you toward a fulfilling post-menopausal journey, incorporating the insights shared in the book. Answer honestly using the bracketed options "Often," "Sometimes," or "Rarely."

Personal Growth & Development:

1. I actively seek opportunities for personal and professional growth, embracing change. (Often)
2. I sometimes struggle with accepting the challenges of menopause, but I actively seek support and resources. (Sometimes)
3. I experience anxiety about the future and haven't explored options for personal development. (Rarely)

Workplace Advocacy:

1. I openly communicate my needs and advocate for supportive policies at my workplace. (Often)
2. I hesitate to discuss menopause-related challenges with my employer, fearing stigma or bias. (Sometimes)
3. I haven't explored resources or support systems available within my workplace. (Rarely)

Lifelong Learning:

1. I actively engage in learning new skills and expanding my knowledge base. (Often)
2. I recognize the importance of lifelong learning but haven't actively pursued new skills. (Sometimes)

3. I lack the motivation to learn new things and haven't considered the benefits of lifelong learning. (Rarely)

Creative Expression:

1. I actively explore creative outlets and express myself through various pursuits. (Often)
2. I have creative interests but haven't prioritized exploring them due to other commitments. (Sometimes)
3. I haven't explored creative pursuits and struggle to identify avenues for self-expression. (Rarely)

Global Perspectives:

1. I recognize the impact of cultural perspectives on menopause and seek to learn from diverse experiences. (Often)
2. I have limited knowledge about different cultural perspectives on menopause and haven't explored them. (Sometimes)
3. I hold limited awareness of how social and cultural factors influence experiences of menopause. (Rarely)

Community Building:

1. I actively engage with communities and support networks focused on menopause and women's health. (Often)
2. I recognize the value of community but haven't actively sought out connections with others. (Sometimes)
3. I feel isolated and lack connections with communities addressing menopause and women's health. (Rarely)

Reflection & Action:

1. I identify my strengths and embrace opportunities to leverage them during this transition. (Often)
2. I sometimes struggle to identify my strengths and need guidance in utilizing them effectively. (Sometimes)
3. I lack confidence in my strengths and hesitate to explore opportunities for growth and empowerment. (Rarely)

Remember:

- There are no right or wrong answers. This quiz is a starting point for self-reflection.
- Celebrate your strengths and areas of progress.
- Identify areas where you might benefit from additional resources or support.
- Embark on your post-menopausal journey with confidence and a willingness to learn and grow.
- Remember, you're not alone! Seek out communities and resources to connect with others on this journey.

I hope this quiz empowers you to embrace your post-menopausal journey with a sense of growth, connection, and self-discovery.

Disclaimer: This quiz is intended for informational purposes only and does not constitute medical advice. Please consult with your healthcare provider for personalized recommendations.

NOTES:

_____

_____

_____

Conclusion

As we conclude our transformative journey through the maze of menopause, let's take a moment to bask in the wisdom we've gained and the empowerment we've fostered together.

The goal of this book was to offer you the WELLNESS framework—the map to reclaim control over your body and your life.

- **W**isdom in Menopause: Understanding the Three Master Hormones
- **E**xploring the Menopausal Symphony of Symptoms
- **L**iving Well: Diet and Nutrition in Menopause
- **L**eaping Forward: Physical Activity and Exercise for Menopause
- **N**urturing Health: Holistic and Alternative Therapies
- **E**mbracing Community: Building a Support Network for Menopause
- **S**taying Balanced: Menopause and Mental Well-being
- **S**tepping into the Future: Navigating Post-Menopause

Throughout our journey, we delved into the intricate details of hormones, uncovering the secrets of estrogen, progesterone, and testosterone, the three main controllers of this phase. We've navigated through the range of symptoms with strength and elegance.

Guided by a whole body wellness approach, we investigated the world of healthy eating and the importance of hydration, understanding the amazing impact of nourishing our bodies with good food and pure water. We also jumped into the world of exercise, uncovering the incredible power of movement in making us feel better both physically and mentally.

Our journey didn't stop there. We explored the world of holistic and alternative therapies, uncovering how acupuncture, herbal remedies, and mindfulness practices can enhance traditional treatments. Along the way, we formed connections and created a supportive community, understanding the importance of sharing experiences and learning from each other.

We talked, at length, about the importance of prioritizing mental well-being. We discovered savvy strategies for staying centered, from embracing self-care and stress-busting techniques to seeking expert help when necessary. As we approach the post-menopausal phase, we are armed with the know-how and confidence to glide through it with ease.

We were reminded of the power of solidarity and support. We discovered the immeasurable value of leaning on our menopausal sisters, finding solace and strength in their shared experiences. Together, we embraced this phase not as an end but as a renewal—a chance to redefine ourselves and embrace the possibilities that lie ahead.

So, my fellow adventurers, I challenge you to carry forth the torch of wisdom and empowerment. Share your newfound insights with others, speak your truth, and break the stigma of silence surrounding menopause. Let your voice be heard, and together, let's empower the next generation of women to navigate this journey with grace and resilience.

I invite you to leave a review and share your thoughts on how this book has enriched your journey. Your feedback will help guide future travelers through menopause, ensuring that no woman faces this phase alone.

Thank you for embarking on this voyage with me, and may your path ahead be illuminated with love, happiness, and boundless empowerment.

Others Want to Hear Your Story

We are living in a unique time; one in which our thoughts, opinions, and views matter greatly… one in which the voices of everyday people are far more influential than that of celebrities and advertising media.

This book was designed to help women navigate their journey through menopause in an informed, strategic way. My hope is for readers across the globe to take the reins of their health and well-being, so they are ready to take on any challenges that menopause might throw their way. A few words from you, gentle reader, can help make that happen.

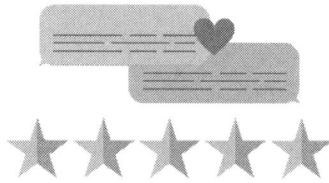

Thank you so much for your support. May you emerge from menopause stronger, more confident, and with a clearer roadmap for a happier, healthier life.

Scan the QR code to leave your review.

References

9 top tips to boost your mood & resilience during menopause in winter [Post]. (2023, November 23). LinkedIn. https://www.linkedin.com/pulse/9-top-tips-boost-your-mood-resilience-during-menopause-fl03e

12 of the best essential oils for menopause—how to naturally balance. (2023, February 4). *Quiet Blue.* https://www.quiet-blue.com/blogs/news/12-of-the-best-essential-oils-for-menopause-how-to-naturally-balance-your-hormones

Ackerman, C. (2017, January 18). *22 mindfulness exercises, techniques & activities for adults (+ pdf).* PositivePsychology.com. https://positivepsychology.com/mindfulness-exercises-techniques-activities

AMC Team. (n.d.). *How omega-3 can provide relief for menopausal symptoms.* Australian Menopause Centre. https://www.menopausecentre.com.au/information-centre/articles/how-omega-3-can-provide-relief-for-menopausal-symptoms

Angelou, M. (n.d.). *Maya Angelou quotes.* Goodreads. https://www.goodreads.com/quotes/67256-we-all-should-know-that-diversity-makes-for-a-rich

Aninye, I. O., Laitner, M. H., & Chinnappan, S. (2021). Menopause preparedness: perspectives for patient, provider, and policymaker consideration. *Menopause, 28*(10), 1186–1191. https://doi.org/10.1097/gme.0000000000001819

Atkins, A. (2023, April 14). *Menopause apps you should know about.* Everyday Health. https://www.everydayhealth.com/menopause/menopause-apps-you-should-know-about

Bartosch, J. (2023, April 24). *Why am I gaining weight so fast during menopause? And will hormone therapy help?* UChicago Medicine. https://www.uchicagomedicine.org/forefront/womens-health-articles/menopause-weight-gain-hormone-therapy

Barraclough, A. (2023, October 10). *How gut health can support symptoms of the menopause.* Women's Health. https://www.womenshealthmag.com/uk/food/a45481427/menopause-and-gut-health

Bioidentical hormones. (2022, April 15). Cleveland Clinic. https://my.clevelandclinic.org/health/treatments/15660-bioidentical-hormones

Breus, Dr. M. (2018, August 2). 7 natural supplements that can help with sleep and menopause. *Psychology Today.* https://www.psychologytoday.com/us/blog/sleep-newzzz/201808/7-natural-supplements-can-help-sleep-and-menopause

Brown, J. (2001). *H. Jackson Brown, Jr. quotes.* BrainyQuote. https://www.brainyquote.com/quotes/h_jackson_brown_jr_382774

Byzak, A. (2017, September 7). *Menopause: What to expect and when to seek help.* Tri-

City Medical Center. https://www.tricitymed.org/2017/09/menopause-expect-seek-help

Cardio training during the menopause. (2022, August 2). Fitnesslab.fit. https://fitnesslab.fit/cardio-training-during-the-menopause

Chan. (2020, September 14). *Mindful eating.* The Nutrition Source. https://www.hsph.harvard.edu/nutritionsource/mindful-eating

Cirino, E. (2023, October 24). *Tips for menopausal hot flashes and night sweats.* Healthline. https://www.healthline.com/health/menopause/hot-flashes-at-night

Cohen, M. (2022, July 26). *7 best exercises to do during menopause, according to experts.* Good Housekeeping. https://www.goodhousekeeping.com/health/fitness/g40476189/menopause-exercises

Cotsen, B. (2018). *Counselling for menopause: Therapy for emotional support.* https://citytherapyrooms.co.uk/counselling-therapy-london/emotional-support-counselling-for-menopause

Crossett, S. (2023, September 18). *Managing menopause symptoms: The role of life coaching* [Post]. LinkedIn. https://www.linkedin.com/pulse/managing-menopause-symptoms-role-life-coaching-crossett-ba-hons-iphm-opade

Deepeshwar, S., Tanwar, M., Kavuri, V., & Budhi, R. B. (2018). Effect of yoga based lifestyle intervention on patients with knee osteoarthritis: A randomized controlled trial. *Frontiers in psychiatry, 9.* https://doi.org/10.3389/fpsyt.2018.00180

Does mindfulness help with menopause? (n.d.). Balance Menopause. https://www.balance-menopause.com/menopause-library/does-mindfulness-help-with-menopause

Donsky, A. (2024). *Family support during menopause.* Morphus. https://wearemorphus.com/blogs/relationships/family-support-during-menopause

Dunleavy, B. (2022, July 20). *9 tricks to battle memory loss in menopause.* Everyday Health. https://www.everydayhealth.com/menopause-pictures/tricks-to-battle-memory-loss-in-menopause.aspx

Evans, T. (2021, February 10). *Managing menopause part 4: Vitamins & minerals.* Health Stand Nutrition Counseling. https://www.healthstandnutrition.com/managing-menopause-vitamins-and-minerals

Ferguson, S. J. (2016, July 6). *Women and education: Qualifications, skills and technology.* Statistics Canada. https://www150.statcan.gc.ca/n1/pub/89-503-x/2015001/article/14640-eng.htm

Gordon, D. (2021, July 13). 73% of women don't treat their menopause symptoms, new survey shows. *Forbes.* https://www.forbes.com/sites/debgordon/2021/07/13/73-of-women-dont-treat-their-menopause-symptoms-new-survey-shows

Harrison, L. (2023, August 21). *Unleashing your potential post-menopause: time for new goals and new beginnings.* Loliya Harrison. https://loliyaharrison.co.uk/unleashing-your-potential-post-menopause-time-for-new-goals-and-new-beginnings

Haskey, J. (2023, April 6). *Staying hydrated*. The Menopause Charity. https://www. themenopausecharity.org/2023/04/06/staying-hydrated

Henderson, E. (2022, July 20). *Telehealth may be a great way for treating some menopause symptoms*. News-Medical. https://www.news-medical.net/news/20220720/ Telehealth-may-be-a-great-way-for-treating-some-menopause-symptoms.aspx

Henry Ford Health Staff. (n.d.). What to eat or not during menopause. *Henry Ford Health*. https://www.henryford.com/blog/2019/03/what-to-eat-or-not-during-menopause

Herbs for menopause. (2024). Meno Martha International Menopause Directory. https://menomartha.com/health-topic/herbs-for-menopause

Hill, A. (2020, September 30). *10 herbs and supplements for menopause*. Healthline. https://www.healthline.com/nutrition/menopause-herbs

Hippocrates. (n.d.). *Hippocrates quotes*. The Quotations Page. http://www.quotation spage.com/quote/24180.html

Hodgkinson, K. (2023a). Latest gut health research: IBS causes & symptoms revealed. *Dr. Vegan*. https://drvegan.com/blogs/articles/latest-gut-health-research-ibs-causes-and-symptoms

Hodgkinson, K. (2023b). How menopause affects gut health. *Dr. Vegan*. https:// drvegan.com/blogs/articles/how-gut-health-changes-during-menopause

How to combat menopausal brain fog. (2022, December 1). *Health Direct*. https:// www.healthdirect.gov.au/blog/how-to-combat-menopausal-brain-fog

The importance of strength training in peri-menopause and beyond. (2023, February 6). Promensil. https://promensil.co.uk/the-importance-of-strength-training-in-peri-menopause-and-beyond

Israel, P. (n.d.). *Treating menopausal symptoms with massage, acupressure and acupuncture*. Peaceful Spirit Massage and Wellness Centers. https://www.bestmassageintuc son.com/category-s/195.htm

James, M. (2017, October 18). *7 ways to unleash your creativity in menopause*. Women's Health Network. https://www.womenshealthnetwork.com/menopause-and-perimenopause/seven-ways-to-help-your-creativity-catch-fire-during-menopause

Johnson, P. (2020, August 5). Estrogen hormone replacement & cortisol levels. *HerKare*. https://herkare.com/blog/estrogen-hormone-replacement-cortisol-levels

Johnson, T. (2022, November 20). *11 supplements for menopause*. WebMD. https:// www.webmd.com/menopause/ss/slideshow-menopause

Junggren, M. (2023, January 3). Try strength training and other exercises to reduce "meno belly." *Bonafide*. https://hellobonafide.com/blogs/news/try-strength-training-and-other-exercises-to-reduce-menopause-belly

Karalis, S., Karalis, T., Foteini Malakoudi, Ioannis Thanasas, Kleisiari, A. S., Zacharoula Tzeli, Papavasiliou, E., & Karalis, D. (2023). Role of phytoestrogen in menopausal women with depressive symptoms: A consecutive case series study. *Cureus.* https://doi.org/10.7759/cureus.37222

Kelly, G. (2016, April 13). *10 ways to build resilience.* HCPLive. https://www.hcplive.com/view/10-ways-to-build-resilience

Kelly. (2023, July 17). *The power of support: Building a community for menopausal women.* NewsBreak Original. https://original.newsbreak.com/@kelly-1602313/3092106486525-the-power-of-support-building-a-community-for-menopausal-women

Ko, J., & Park, Y.-M. (2021). Menopause and the loss of skeletal muscle mass in women. *Iranian journal of public health, 50*(2). https://doi.org/10.18502/ijph.v50i2.5362

Letts, R. (n.d.). Mood changes during menopause—does what you eat make a difference? *Health & Her.* https://healthandher.com/blogs/expert-advice/mood-changes-during-menopause-does-what-you-eat-make-a-difference

Lin, Y.-Y., & Lee, S.-D. (2018). Cardiovascular benefits of exercise training in postmenopausal hypertension. *International journal of molecular sciences, 19*(9), 2523. https://doi.org/10.3390/ijms19092523

Luque, M. (2020, June 24). *Menopause menu: Probiotics.* New Moves. https://www.fitnessinmenopause.com/blog/menopause-menu-probiotics

Macros for menopause weight loss: A comprehensive guide. (2023, April 19). Golden Leaf Health Center. https://goldenleafhc.com/mastering-macros-for-menopause-weight-loss-a-comprehensive-guide

The many benefits of lifelong learning. (n.d.). Walden University. https://www.waldenu.edu/programs/resource/the-many-benefits-of-lifelong-learning

Matsui, S., Yasui, T., Tani, A., Kunimi, K., Uemura, H., Yamamoto, S., Kuwahara, A., Matsuzaki, T., & Irahara, M. (2013). Associations of estrogen and testosterone with insulin resistance in pre- and postmenopausal women and postmenopausal women with hormone therapy. *International journal of endocrinology and metabolism, 11*(2). https://doi.org/10.5812/ijem.5333

Mayo Clinic Staff. (2019a). *The reality of menopause weight gain.* Mayo Clinic. https://www.mayoclinic.org/healthy-lifestyle/womens-health/in-depth/menopause-weight-gain/art-20046058

Mayo Clinic Staff. (2019b, June 21). *Mediterranean diet for heart health.* Mayo Clinic. https://www.mayoclinic.org/healthy-lifestyle/nutrition-and-healthy-eating/in-depth/mediterranean-diet/art-20047801

Mayo Clinic Staff. (2022, November 2). *Low-glycemic index diet: What's behind the claims?* Mayo Clinic. https://www.mayoclinic.org/healthy-lifestyle/nutrition-and-healthy-eating/in-depth/low-glycemic-index-diet/art-20048478

Mayo Clinic Staff. (2023, May 25). *Perimenopause.* Mayo Clinic. https://www.mayoclinic.org/diseases-conditions/perimenopause/symptoms-causes/syc-20354666

McKenna, D. W. (2023, March 7). *Chiropractic can help with menopause symptoms.*

Braincore Therapy and Wellness. https://www.dutchessbraincore.com/chiro practic-care/chiropractic-can-help-with-menopause-symptoms

Menopause and weight. (n.d.). Better Health. https://www.betterhealth.vic.gov.au/ health/conditionsandtreatments/menopause-and-weight-gain

Menopause in different cultures. (2023, February 27). Women's Health Network. https://www.womenshealthnetwork.com/menopause-and-perimenopause/ menopause-in-different-cultures

Menopause. (n.d.). Mount Sinai Health System. https://www.mountsinai.org/ health-library/report/menopause

Migala, J. (2023, January 23). *5 potential health benefits of guided imagery meditation.* EverydayHealth. https://www.everydayhealth.com/integrative-health/poten tial-health-benefits-of-guided-imagery-meditation

Montgomery, T. (2023, June 30). *How menopause can affect your career progression* [Post]. LinkedIn. https://www.linkedin.com/pulse/how-menopause-can- affect-your-career-progression-tracey-montgomery

Mukherjee, A. (2023, May 18). *Thyroid and menopause article.* British Thyroid Foun- dation. https://www.btf-thyroid.org/thyroid-and-menopause-article

Muldoon, N. (n.d.). *Reflexology for the menopause.* Reflexology in Tring. https://www. sleepingbeautytherapies.co.uk/reflexology/reflexology-menopause

Mullin, E. (2023, May 2). *The secrets of aging are hidden in your ovaries.* Wired. https://www.wired.com/story/aging-menopause-longevity

Newton, K., & Snyder, L. (2021, April 29). *Tai Chi and Qigong.* My Menoplan. https://mymenoplan.org/tai-chi

Office on Women's Health: https://www.womenshealth.gov/menopause

Osteoporosis—causes. (2017, October 23). NHS. https://www.nhs.uk/conditions/ osteoporosis/causes

Pass It On. "Helping Others." Accessed March 18, 2024. https://www.passiton. com/inspirational-quotes/7628-one-of-the-greatest-things-you-can-do-to-help

Payne, J. (2024). *Can menopause cause depression?* Johns Hopkins Medicine. https:// www.hopkinsmedicine.org/health/wellness-and-prevention/can-menopause- cause-depression

Perimenopause. (2021). Cleveland Clinic. https://my.clevelandclinic.org/health/ diseases/21608-perimenopause

Platzman-Weinstock, C. (2023, January 4). All about boundary setting: why do it and how to get better at it. EverydayHealth. https://www.everydayhealth. com/emotional-health/all-about-boundary-setting-why-do-it-and-how-to-get- better-at-it

Postmenopause. (2021, May 10). Cleveland Clinic. https://my.clevelandclinic.org/ health/diseases/21837-postmenopause

Railton, D. (2023, February 15). *What is the link between menopause and anxiety?* MedicalNewsToday. https://www.medicalnewstoday.com/articles/317552

Reiki for menopause energy healing sessions. (2023, April 12). Menopause Health-

Matters.   https://menopausehealthmatters.co.uk/our-services/reiki-energy-healing

Santos-Longhurst, A. (2018, August 30). *Why is oxytocin known as the "love hormone"? and 11 other FAQs.* Healthline. https://www.healthline.com/health/love-hormone

Schwenkhagen, A. (2007). Hormonal changes in menopause and implications on sexual health. *The journal of sexual medicine, 4*, 220–226. https://doi.org/10.1111/j.1743-6109.2007.00448.x

Sleep problems and menopause: What can I do? (2021, September 30). National Institute on Aging. https://www.nia.nih.gov/health/menopause/sleep-problems-and-menopause-what-can-i-do

Spencer, C. (n.d.). *Staying healthy in postmenopausal life.* My Menopause Centre. https://www.mymenopausecentre.com/knowledge/life-after-menopause

Spritzler, F. (2021, May 12). How to lose weight around menopause (and keep it off). Healthline. https://www.healthline.com/nutrition/lose-weight-in-menopause

Stills, S. S. (2013, October 28). *How to avoid insulin resistance.* Women's Health Network. https://www.womenshealthnetwork.com/blood-sugar/how-to-avoid-insulin-resistance

Suni, E. (2023, November 8). *How to design the ideal bedroom for sleep.* Sleep Foundation. https://www.sleepfoundation.org/bedroom-environment/how-to-design-the-ideal-bedroom-for-sleep

The National Institute on Aging: https://www.nia.nih.gov/health/topics/menopause

The North American Menopause Society: https://www.menopause.org/

Top 10 menopause forums in 2024. (2024, February 17). FeedSpot for Forum Lists and Online Message Boards. https://forums.feedspot.com/menopause_forums

Top 10 things to know about the second edition of the physical activity guidelines for Americans. (2021, August 25). Health.gov. https://health.gov/our-work/nutrition-physical-activity/physical-activity-guidelines/current-guidelines/top-10-things-know

University of South Wales Prifysgol De Cymru. "10 Facts about the Menopause." October 16, 2020. https://health.research.southwales.ac.uk/health-research-news/10-facts-about-menopause/

Verona, T. (2022, July 13). *7 best menopause teas of 2023.* Hello Again. https://helloagainproducts.com/2022/07/13/menopause-tea-reviews

Villaverde Gutiérrez, C., Torres Luque, G., Ábalos Medina, G. M., Argente del Castillo, M. J., Guisado, I. M., Guisado Barrilao, R., & Ramírez Rodrigo, J. (2012). Influence of exercise on mood in postmenopausal women. *Journal of clinical nursing, 21*(7–8), 923–928. https://doi.org/10.1111/j.1365-2702.2011.03972.x

Vroomen, M. (2020, May 29). *Understanding and dealing with hot flashes*. Healthline. https://www.healthline.com/health/menopause/understanding-hot-flashes

Walsh, K. (2022, October 4). *7 bedtime snacks to support your metabolism*. EatingWell. https://www.eatingwell.com/article/291888/bedtime-snacks-to-support-your-metabolism

WebMD Editorial Contributors. (2023a, April 7). *The emotional roller coaster of menopause*. WebMD. https://www.webmd.com/menopause/emotional-roller-coaster

WebMD Editorial Contributors. (2023b, July 14). *Learning to relax during menopause*. WebMD. https://www.webmd.com/menopause/learning-relax-during-menopause

Weiss, C. (2022, October 25). *Menopause awareness and education should start earlier in life*. Mayo Clinic News Network. https://newsnetwork.mayoclinic.org/discussion/menopause-awareness-and-education-should-start-earlier-in-life

What is menopause? (2021, September 30). National Institute on Aging. https://www.nia.nih.gov/health/menopause/what-menopause

Wilkinson, Dr. L. (2022, April 22). *Stress and menopause*. Stella. https://www.onstella.com/the-latest/long-term-health/stress-and-menopause

Yazdkhasti, M., Keshavarz, M., Khoei, E. M., Hosseini, A., ESmaeilzadeh, S., Pebdani, M. A., & Jafarzadeh, H. (2012). The effect of support group method on quality of life in post-menopausal women. *Iranian journal of public health*, *41*(11), 78–84. https://www.ncbi.nlm.nih.gov/pmc/articles/PMC3521890

Yeager, S. (2022a, May 30). What's the best diet for menopausal brain health? *Feisty Menopause*. https://www.feistymenopause.com/blog/best-diet-for-menopausal-brain-health

Yeager, S. (2023b, August 29). How to keep your menopausal joints healthy and happy. *Feisty Menopause*. https://www.feistymenopause.com/blog/keep-menopausal-joints-happy-and-healthy

Yeager, S. (2023c, September 3). How to manage inflammation during menopause. *Feisty Menopause*. https://www.feistymenopause.com/blog/Manage-Inflammation-During-Menopause

Yoga, meditation and the menopause. (2019, December 9). Menopause Treatment. https://menopausetreatment.co.uk/yoga-meditation-and-the-menopause

Yüksel, O., Ateş, M., Kızıldağ, S., Yüce, Z., Koç, B., Kandiş, S., Güvendi, G., Karakılıç, A., Gümüş, H., & Uysal, N. (2019). Regular aerobic voluntary exercise increased oxytocin in female mice: The cause of decreased anxiety and increased empathy-like behaviors. *Balkan medical journal*, *36*(5), 257–262. https://doi.org/10.4274/balkanmedj.galenos.2019.2018.12.87

Printed in Great Britain
by Amazon